UNDER THE DESK

REALIZING YOUR NEW SELF

AN INTIMATE STORY OF STROKE RECOVERY

BRYAN MARKS

Printed in the United States of America.

ISBN: 978-1-958032-29-9

This book is a work of non-fiction.

Illustrations and cover design by Tom Garber

Book formatting by Jennifer Gunn

Sandi Huddleston-Edwards, Publisher

Published by Here I Am Publishing, LLC
780 Monterrosa Drive
Myrtle Beach, South Carolina 29572

HERE I AM
PUBLISHING, LLC

DEDICATION

I dedicate this book to my loving daughters, Jennifer, Maura, and Sara, whom I affectionately call my Girlies. I am a truly blessed father who God gave me you three in my life. Your grandma Vivian said her greatest accomplishments in life were her family. THANK YOU for being my three greatest accomplishments in life. I love you, Girlies, more than you can possibly imagine! Each of you are strong, accomplished, and LOVING souls to all you touch. I am so proud of you, Girlies.

To my wife Abbey, thank you for your endless energy in taking care of our family and researching everything about healthcare for us. You worked tirelessly to make me comfortable at the hospitals, for my return home, and ALL through my recovery and journey in life. Abbey, you are always *there* for us. Thank you for wearing so many hats simultaneously as you look out for us. You are the safe one to go to for EVERYTHING. Thank you for being you. As we had inscribed on our wedding bands, Forever Yours.

To my brothers, Edward, Alan, and Eldon, and sisters-in-law, Ann and Ruth. Thank you for your love, encouragement, care, and advice then and now. Big brothers and sisters make life easier. We hardly say we love each other enough, but it is felt. I learn a great deal from my big brothers, none more important than their life perspectives, rationality, and calmness in the heat of a moment. Their humor is not too shabby either! Thank you for all you taught me and for letting me cry when we play chess.

To my Uncle Solomon for whom I would give anything to have ANOTH-ER shared moment of time. I love you and miss your gentle demeanor, physical presence, and baritone voice. You confirmed you are always beside me in some fashion. Your life on earth was admired by so many and continues to live on within us and God's afterlife. "Everything is gonna be alllllllllriiiighttttt." I look forward to being with you again, just not anytime soon!

To family members who have passed on to their eternal bliss, they are certainly not forgotten, as their love, teachings, and inspirations remain in my heart and remind me of them every day. Each of you has provided me with wonderful opportunities in life, and your legacies to provide each new family generation greater opportunities have been taught and shared. I visit and hug you all in my heart and mind every day.

To Doctor Steven Kittner, his neurology team, and ALL the doctors, nurses, technicians, hospital staff, and rehabilitation therapists at every hospital, too many to name, who saved my life, then cared for me with a supportive, unwavering dedication to help me recover and get my life back in order. Doctor Kittner had a patient with multiple diagnostic challenges, and he and his team remained faithful in their care for multiple months, overseeing my healthcare. Because of everyone's care, I lead a very good life again. They saved my life!

A heartfelt thank you to Howard County General Hospital, University of Maryland Hospital/Stroke Center, Sinai Hospital of Baltimore, Humanim Rehabilitation, and the Brain Injury Association of America and ALL its charters in the United States. Their services and staff will never be forgotten. I give each of them my forever gratitude for caring for me and helping me.

TABLE OF CONTENTS

FOREWORD

Every person is on an unpredictable journey. No one expects to have a stroke in the prime of life as a young adult. When this happens to someone, they must face and deal with a cascade of physical, cognitive, emotional, and social changes. Not only they, but their family and loved ones, are also enmeshed in the changes resulting from the stroke.

Though the experience of every person and family after a stroke is different, there are certain commonalities. Bryan Marks has written an insightful and unflinchingly honest account of his post-stroke journey that would be useful to any person or family dealing with the sequelae of a stroke, particularly those in their young adult years. He describes the physical changes that he met with grit and determination and, more importantly, the changes to his sense of identity and behavior that were even more challenging to him and his family than the physical changes. He depicts the grieving process at the loss of his old, pre-stroke self and shame at his inability to prevent negative interactions with his wife and children in the early years after his stroke. Yet, ultimately, this is an inspiring story as he heals emotionally with the love and support of his family.

All stroke survivors and their families, as well as their physicians, would benefit from reading this book to gain a greater awareness and sensitivity to the "invisible wounds" caused by stroke.

—**Steven J. Kittner,** MD, MPH
Professor of Neurology
Distinguished University Professor
University of Maryland School of Medicine.

INTRODUCTION

The book entitled, *Under the Desk, Realizing Your New Self, An Intimate Story of Stroke Recovery*, was inspired by my daughter Jennifer. I learned much later she used to hide under our office desk as a young child to cope with the angry home environment immediately after my life-altering stroke.

My daughters, Jennifer, Maura, and Sara, who I affectionately call My Girlies, and my wife, Abbey, were affected by my subsequent ramped-up verbal anger upon returning home from rehabilitation hospitals. I struggled to understand that a *new me* evolved immediately post-stroke. At the start of my healing journey, I did not accept my brain had dramatically changed, let alone produced an emotionally ugly personality within me. I call this my hidden disability, not recognizing a *new me* evolved and the radical negative personality changes that temporarily overcame me.

The highly personal stories in this book are meant to showcase the struggles of personality change post-stroke for readers, caregivers, or those in medical professions assisting a stroke survivor or a brain-injured patient without drawing on self-pity or a woe-is-me projection of attitude. I am a very fortunate and grateful survivor whose only motivation in sharing such personal stories is to help other survivors learn and cope with their potential personality and behavior struggles post-stroke. I believe books regarding stroke tend to focus on the more common subtopics, with few focusing on the least common subtopic of personality change other than to generalize things as mood swings or something else. In 2005, the year of my stroke event, I found limited readings specific to personality changes other than personality changes may be a byproduct of stroke.

At the lowest point of my recovery, I was desperate to learn how other survivors experiencing negative personality changes overcame their angry behavior. I searched for books, articles, journals, pamphlets, and spoke to other stroke survivors in hopes of comprehending my *new me*. Unfortunately, nearly everything I read addressed other topics of stroke, such as how the brain functions and heals itself, or provided medical jargon and definitions centering on the more common areas of recovery, such as cognitive, physical, speech, and occupational rehabilitation.

A nurse who regularly facilitates a stroke support group I attend now thought there may not be many published research studies specifically relating to survivors who suffer from personality change because those within study groups may not be entirely forthcoming on their struggles for fear of potential humiliation, vulnerability to judgment, and not wanting to speak of such a difficult time in their lives. I respected her answer. My family and I certainly did not want to go through our own experiences, let alone re-live them through writing this book, which presents personal accounts to tell a story.

There is now an abundance of knowledgeable information regarding stroke and its subtopics as new research, data, and proven treatments have recently become available since as early as 2015.

At the time of my stroke in 2005, there was still so much for the medical community to learn and understand about stroke and brain injuries, especially how a person's personality may be affected. Even with today's knowledge, experts are still learning how the brain can change who we are as a person.

Dr. Andy Josephson from the University of California at San Francisco, Department of Medicine, presented a seminar entitled, "Stroke 2023, A Change has Come and is Still Coming," which may be viewed on *YouTube*. The seminar addressed exciting current advances and shifts in the management of acute strokes, presenting new data and new directions for stroke research.

I was extremely fortunate to have Dr. Kittner, an expert on stroke, and his neurology team oversee my healthcare and treatment at the University of Maryland Medical Center immediately upon arrival. Dr. Kittner and his team helped save my life and his work and devotion to stroke research has undoubtedly saved the lives of countless others. My greatest hope is this book makes a positive difference in your life and serves as an insightful tool for you, your loved ones, family, caregivers, or those in the healthcare profession by providing perspectives and insights from a survivor's experience. I made a great deal of mistakes and created damage on my journey toward trying to *right the ship* post-stroke as my family and I struggled with my *new self*.

I hope this book shines some light on the potential change of personality within a survivor AND maybe, just maybe, inspires further research, conversation, and the desire to delve deeper into this area of stroke damage. My Uncle Solomon had the strength to find something good in something terrible. I hope I have accomplished the same by writing my family's story. In this book, I include **Sidebars** for the purposes of complementing and adding context to the main topic. Sometimes using a Sidebar to mix in a dash of humor. After all, "Laughter is indeed the best medicine!"

Remember: You are not alone in your journey.

PROLOGUE

I was forty-two when I had my stroke. On the day of my stroke, which was a Saturday, June 18, 2005, I woke up at six in the morning, feeling great, ready to run a calculated eleven-mile course with a running partner in preparation for completing another marathon. The early morning showed promise of being an all-around beautiful day filled with bright sunshine, few clouds, and a slow cool breeze. By all accounts, I was healthy from doctors' perspectives, completing marathons and feeling proud of my fitness regimen of different exercises, including bike riding and weightlifting. My goal was to stave off middle age for a bit longer. I also looked very forward to vacationing in Alaska with my wife, Abbey, on our first cruise, leaving in just four days. I envisioned our time together filled with laughter, holding hands, dancing, and looking at Abbey's beautiful eyes and smile, which would complement the breathtaking Alaskan landscape and wildlife. The totality of being together was an exciting start to my day!

After completing the morning training run, I felt great and could have continued a little further as I was working off a runner's high. However, my running partner and I decided it would be wiser to cool down, hydrate, and converse about the day's plans and the week ahead. The end of our route was at my house. *So soon,* I thought. I would satisfy my hankering for scrambled eggs, toast, and an energy drink for breakfast. I was truly excited to begin a planned weekend of hedonism since my family was enjoying some R&R at the family lake house a few hours away.

I could put off showering to dive into breakfast first as I had no immediate responsibilities other than to myself. My buddy, Louis, would join me in the evening for a movie and our usual comedic repartee and bantering. I met Louis in college, so he knew me well; most importantly, he knew me before my stroke. It is said that the older you become, the more you need the people who knew you when you were younger. This saying has proven particularly true for me as I desire to have those who knew me before my stroke around me because they easily recognize the total sum of who I am and the true, kind person I am.

My running partner and I called it a "morning" soon after chatting and drinking water. About four minutes after he left, I had the beginnings of my stroke. At first, I thought the symptoms were simply a form of dehydration, so I tried drinking more fluids but was unable to swallow. Every intake of water was now dribbling down my shirt. Moments later, I felt violently dizzy and nauseous and HAD to put myself on the kitchen floor for safety. I never experienced anything like this, so I did not know what was happening. A stroke never entered my thoughts, especially since I initially responded well to my environment. Besides, I was a young man, and I thought healthy, having recently passed stringent medical checkups with my private physician and those required by the medics at work. *So, what could be seriously wrong?*

I began crawling out of the kitchen sliding glass door that led to the backyard, knowing I was going to violently vomit soon and did not want to do so inside the house and then have to clean up, further complicating my day! Plus, my neighbor and good friend, Paul, was working outside in his side yard. I thought if I were in trouble, he would assist me. In hindsight, crawling outside was a blessing as he had to call for medical assistance, and an ambulance arrived within moments. At this point, I no longer needed the ambulance for my health; I just needed to get away from Paul's funny antics and teasing about how awful I looked. He stated that I took him away from yard work and house chores. However, I suspect he didn't want to do the toiling anyway. I was an excuse for delaying his busy day.

I thanked Paul for being outside at the perfect moment to provide timely assistance, shuddering to think what could have happened had he not seen me lying on the walkout landing. To this day, we joke about my needing his assistance and how I should forever wash and wax his cars as payback for his good deed.

Still aware of my surroundings and the fact that I had not eaten breakfast or showered, I felt I only needed time to rehydrate and simply asked the ambulance medics to please give me fluids through my veins to speed up my recovery. Unfortunately, my only choices were to refuse help, go to the community hospital, or listen to Paul lightheartedly *mother* me by telling me what was best. I opted for the hospital. Still in good spirits, I joked with the ambulance crew about never having an ambulance ride and asked them to please turn on the lights and sirens so I could experience the royal treatment of riding in style and quickly getting treated.

The emergency department became a scene you watched on television or in movies, with the medics calling out stats and the scrambling of varying hospital staff to provide immediate care. I was optimistic I would be out of the hospital in a couple of hours after my body was refueled from lost critical fluids. Until then, this event was a minor holding pattern to my planned hedonistic day. My good-natured attitude was, *Heck, I might as well enjoy the hospital staff's warm, welcoming, and over- the-top gracious attention as if I were their only patient.* The staff's genuine smiles and care were warmly appreciated, given what I thought would be a minor visit and treatment.

Who knew what was to happen next?

NO ONE KNOWS

It's so hard to explain to people
Why my life is like it is now.
I just say it's a long story
Because it's hard to explain how.

How my life changed forever
Within the moments of a day
When a tragic event had taken place
While me, my mom, and my sisters were away.

Most people don't even know about it
Because it's a huge secret that I keep.
I try not to tell them unless it's necessary
So, they don't know that I smile less than I weep.

When I am with friends, I try to be happy
Because I hide my pain deep down inside
Which prevents them from knowing
About my whole other life that I have momentarily set aside.

My whole other life
Is a whole different story
Full of roller coaster-like hardships
But don't worry, it never got gory.

No one knows
Who I am when they are not looking
The person I become when I am at home
Where more and more secrets are cooking.

No one knows about my whole other life
The one I hide in the locked walls of my brain
Not even my family.
No one knows the secrets that I refrain.

—**Maura Marks** (Bryan's daughter)

("No One Knows" I wrote about pretending everything was okay when I was at school or with my friends, but deep down, I was carrying the burden of the uncertainty of our home life.)

CHAPTER 1:
THE DAY OF MY STROKE

Doctors and nurses conducting the triage placed me in a curtained-off section of the emergency room while they observed my symptoms. Since I complained of dehydration and was not displaying glaring evidence of a stroke, I was initially treated as such as they hung fluid bags and inserted needles into my veins. Shortly after the initial triage and now alone behind the curtains, I became a bit nervous, realizing different symptoms were beginning. The left side of my body became numb. My vision slowly became clouded, then dark. I felt weaker and much dizzier. I remained mostly calm until I had difficulty *staying in the moment*, fading in and out of reality, now feeling helpless and scared. I wanted to yell out for help but had trouble raising my voice above a whisper. Even while slurring the words, I tried to call out.

I did not think anyone would hear or see me through the small gap in the curtain sections, so I contemplated dropping to the floor and crawling out from underneath, figuring the fall could not hurt any worse than I was already feeling. I ended up panicky, waving my right arm at a passing doctor, nurse, or staff administrator who gratefully saw me through the small opening. He or she was acutely aware I was in trouble. Then, I must have blacked out as I missed several minutes of accelerated attention, including being placed on a gurney surrounded by a team of newfound medical friends who were placing more needles in my veins and calling out additional orders.

These new symptoms pointed to a possible stroke, so I was whisked away for scans and imaging, and indeed, initial results proved I was having a severe stroke. Minutes later, upon regaining consciousness, I felt an immediate loss of time. I could not recall the sequence of events and why additional attention was being paid to me. What alarmed me most was that I had forgotten occurrences of seconds ago, or those moments were now hazy at best. I barely remembered a gurney ride through the halls or how I contacted Paul to let him know I would not be home anytime soon. Paul said he had already called Abbey to inform her I was taken to the hospital by ambulance, and I became upset he called because I believed this event was a minor concern. Why alarm her unnecessarily? Months later, I asked Paul questions regarding *that day* as I had no recollection of our conversation. He mentioned I was surly during our phone conversation. (His actual word choice has been edited.)

At this point, emergency room doctors contemplated giving me a typical shot of a Tissue Plasminogen Activator (tPA), which is administered within the first three-to-four hours of stroke symptoms. Its purpose serves as a clot buster for those having an Ischemic stroke—a clot that is blocking blood flow to the brain. But, at that moment, it was not yet possible for any specialist to determine precisely what kind of stroke I was having. Administering the wrong type of medical treatment would have been worse than the stroke itself.

Hospital staff contacted Abbey to inform her I was being treated for what now appeared to be a stroke rather than dehydration and to come to the hospital immediately. She and the Girlies were three-and-a- half hours away, enjoying R&R with her brother's family at the lake house. Abbey began the long drive back home alone. The kids remained behind with family, and while she was enroute, hospital staff called Abbey again, letting her know I was now being processed for transport to another hospital with a specialty stroke unit an hour farther away. The emergency room medical team had quickly recognized I required the next level of expertise in stroke treatment. I fully credit my local hospital staff for saving my life and giving me their very best aid and attention. I know they did everything possible to diagnose, treat, and mitigate the stroke damage as quickly as possible.

- I do not know who or what preparations were made for my transport.
- I do not know if anything was said to me before my departure or during transport to the second hospital.
- I do not even know if I was finally able to ride in royalty having lights and sirens on.
- I do not have a recollection of who greeted me upon arrival at the second hospital and only vaguely recall their triage evaluations as I continued fading in and out of consciousness for an extended time.

I was losing the ability to sequence or make complete sense of events happening to me. I had little control. That is when I simply *let go,* placing all my trust and faith in the hands of those now evaluating me, believing I would continue receiving top-notch care. When able to sustain some sense of reality, which was only for fleeting moments, I was determined to be calm and as lucid as possible to answer or ask questions.

I needed to be calm so as not to panic and exasperate my condition. My *go-to self* uses humor to diffuse situations or as a coping mechanism. During this specific scenario, my attempts at humor relaxed me and hopefully eased those now treating me. I made occasional jokes about my condition with the doctors, nurses, and hospital staff as they conducted additional

A doctor examining me asked, "How long have you had a droopy left eye?"

I replied, "I don't know anything about my left eye." Then I casually mentioned, "But my left testicle hangs much lower than my right" and asked if he would please fix that problem first.

I received a stern reply, "This is no time to joke!"

While I agree my comment was inappropriate, I, at least, smirked because for one second, I found humor in something so scary. I hoped it would stifle my fears. You have to smirk at life sometimes!

evaluations and began ordering brain scans. As critically ill as I was, it was just as critical for me to be lighthearted. I was constantly observed, diagnosed, and treated while Abbey was making the long drive back home, and had now been diverted to the second hospital. She was unsure what she would witness upon arrival. Abbey picked up my brother, Eldon, along the way. When they made it to the hospital, they were informed that the next seventy-two hours would prove crucial in determining my survival and, if I were to survive, how much brain damage occurred, so they could assess my potential quality of life post-stroke. **If I were to survive....**

· • ● • ·

Frequent scans of my brain were necessary because as more blood entered, more swelling occurred. These scans would indicate to doctors what was happening inside my brain and determine their course of action immediately going forward. As the stroke progressed, my left arm and leg began twitching uncontrollably on their own.

"He's experiencing muscle spasticity," a technician called out. My muscles experienced involuntary, rapid contractions, essentially causing them to twitch or jerk unexpectedly. I became absolutely terrified, knowing *perfect* scan images were necessary for the specialists to make intelligent treatment decisions, or I may die. *Somehow, I must stop these violent twitches*. A technician politely suggested lightly tying my left side down to obtain the best imaging results. I agreed. Unfortunately, my left arm and leg now flailed against the Velcro, undoing most of it, so no solid images were obtained to determine exactly where the bleeding was coming from and how swollen my brain was becoming. The primary technician suggested we try again later, but I believed I would die soon without quickly obtaining the best images for the medical team to make educated decisions. *Later* was not a comforting option, so I begged all the technicians near me for another chance. They hesitantly agreed to one final attempt, given that so many other patients needed attention. On this final attempt, a very caring technician gently held my foot for a few seconds before I entered the tube. That very simple, meaningful touch immediately reassured me I was not alone. Her kindness had a HUGE IMPACT on my accepting what was happening.

Once back inside the scanning tube, things became so quiet. My left arm and leg stopped their uncontrolled, violent movements. My breathing became calm, and a tranquil peacefulness rushed over me, allowing the main scan technician to obtain *perfect* images during those few minutes. Then, the very moment I was removed from the tube, my left arm and leg resumed their wild movements, and the peacefulness I had felt dramatically ended.

Were those tranquil few minutes because of my Uncle Solomon, who believed in life after death and God's intervention by sending a loved one to help you in your time of need? I ask these questions to myself, my family, religious friends, clergymen, and anyone who wishes to share their philosophy on life! To this very day, I have no explanation for being able to control myself or feel safe and tranquil during the third scan. I am open-minded enough to believe I had some divine help, but why? Why me? For what purpose? Hopefully, there is a supreme being looking out for us, and we each serve a purpose in life.

I was frightened by what was happening to my body, while ever so thankful useful images were collected! Then I faded out and later woke up in an unfamiliar room, wondering where everybody was. What did they do to me? What is the next course of action? And there were many more questions.

The doctors later determined I suffered a hemorrhagic stroke via left side cerebellar and medullary stroke—a left vertebral artery occlusion. The ruptured vessel bled into areas surrounding my brain, compounded by suffering a Wallenberg's Syndrome, which is a neurological condition caused by my stroke in the brain stem, specifically in an artery that provides blood to the cerebellum. The cerebellum coordinates and regulates muscular activity in the body and is located at the back of the brain, just behind the spinal cord and below the main cerebrum. Generally, the cerebellum is known to control the coordination of voluntary movements, maintain balance and posture, learn motor skills, and control some aspects of language. Therefore, when a stroke occurs in the cerebellum it can damage any or all of these functions. On a *Flint Rehab* posting dated October 13, 2023, it states, "Experiencing a cerebellar stroke is rare, as this specific type accounts for just one to four percent of all strokes." Around one to three percent of people who are rushed to the emergency room for vertigo are having a cerebellar stroke. Since vertigo can be caused by other conditions, this leads to a high misdiagnosis rate, meaning cerebellar stroke is often missed initially. This significantly increases the risk of mortality due to cerebellar stroke and can lead to more severe secondary effects when this goes undiagnosed and untreated.

I initially had severe dysarthria and dysphagia. Dysarthria is defined as difficult or unclear articulation of speech. Wallenberg's Syndrome also affects the nervous system potentially causing hoarseness of the voice. In my case, I suffered total paralysis of my left vocal cord, rendering it permanently dysfunctional. What voice I have after surgeries is indeed hoarse. Dysphagia is associated with swallowing difficulties and appropriately managing food, saliva, and most liquids by mouth. A person with dysphagia is susceptible to frequent choking or aspirating. Soon after my stroke, I developed constant hiccups for multiple days, except while sleeping, and a complete loss of pain and temperature sensations on the right side of my body. In other words, initially, I was a mess and given a one to three percent chance of survival. I experienced secondary cerebellar stroke effects (for definitions, go to the Appendix).

Now, nearly twenty years later, I have returned pain and temperature sensations along with other healings. Today's research proves recovery remains possible even multiple years later. I am nearly twenty years post-stroke and STILL blessed with being able to improve. I like to say I am a testament to all the doctors' and researchers' findings regarding stroke.

Indeed, I am proof of healing multiple years later.

Acute cerebellar ataxia: I experienced sudden jerky left leg movements for nearly nine months post-stroke. They occurred very randomly, mostly when I sat continuously in one position for a few hours. Nothing disturbing, but when my leg decided to jerk, the movement was startling especially since there was not a warning beforehand.

Vertigo: This remains problematic for me as I am dizzy nearly all the time except when finally in bed for the evening.

Difficulty with proprioception: This indeed remains my most difficulty. Recently, I entered a medical building via their automatic sliding glass door. The door was still opening as I misqued and nearly banged into the door as it was still opening. The building receptionist politely held in her laughter until I said, "Go ahead; you've gotta laugh!"

Speech problems: I am slightly more difficult to understand when speaking on the phone versus speaking face-to-face. Occasionally, I'm asked to repeat myself while conversing over the phone.

Eye movement disorders: My nystagmus remains.

CHAPTER 2:
NYSTAGMUS

I developed nystagmus, a condition where the eyes move in rapid, jerky motions, either side to side, up and down, or in circles, making you feel like the world is moving because the brain does not register the eyes are actually moving rather than an object. My nystagmus, I call it jumpy eyes condition, causes my eyes to jump around side to side, so walking, balancing, reading, watching television, or having the normal ability to interpret environmental cues remains challenging. This was discussed in an article of the September/October 2005 issue of *Stroke Connection* magazine. I read everything about stroke that I could get my hands on. "In order to read, track objects, and compensate for body movements, the eyes must move smoothly and accurately. However, after a brain injury, eye movements may become jerky. These symptoms occur because the brain does not recognize it is the eyes that are shaking."

Damage was sustained within my brain stem, thereby causing crossover damage, meaning my right side and left side brain were both affected. Then, to *pile on*, I suffered Horner's Syndrome, also known as Bernard-Horner Syndrome or Oculosympathetic Palsy, a condition affecting the face and eye on one side of the body caused by the disruption of a nerve pathway from the brain to the head and neck. My left eyelid droops, and soon after my stroke, my left eye suffered an eye stroke whereby a fair amount of vision loss occurred. My vision loss, combined with near constant dizziness, complicates the spatial and perceptual deficits driven by my stroke.

I had so much brain damage to occur, it was and still is nearly impossible to sort out what I hope heals first. Balance, dizziness, swallowing, and nausea remain my top four challenges, so sometimes I do not want to open my eyes and move around upon waking up in the morning because many times I cannot feel where I am in space. A doctor called it *proprioception*, which is defined as an awareness of the position and movement of our bodies and where they are located in relation to the surrounding area.

Over the years, I have embarrassed myself more than once post-stroke. The most laughable and memorable moment came when I was speaking face-to-face with a female acquaintance at the local grocery store. After several minutes of conversation, I suddenly became severely dizzy and felt as if I were going to pass out. In complete panic, I hurriedly reached out my hand to grab the grocery shelf, but instantly, realized I had not grabbed the shelf. She said, "Well, that is a much faster way to get to know one another." Whew! I'm glad she had a sense of humor, or that moment could have been dicey!

Depth perception can be confusing and offers several other challenges. I often need assistance going down steps, so I hold someone or use a white-knuckle grip while holding a banister. Climbing steps is easier. How I walk stairs is not pretty, but I can walk them, so I won't complain. Every attempt is therapy. My recovery attitude since day one has consistently been not to shy away from difficult therapies. I just need to be prepared and cautious when accepting them. I do avoid most hiking trails. I know my limits! However, some of the funniest moments come from trying to do simple daily life therapies—**doing life!**

A few weeks after returning home, Jennifer and I went to an indoor mall. I did not use the elevators or escalators, instead choosing the stairs. I was using these moments again as therapy. But, on a whim, I decided to try and use an escalator because I was getting tired and thought I was up for the challenge. I was very cautious, just not prepared since this was a spontaneous decision. I walked onto the platform using my cane and then stared at the rising escalator stairs, trying to time the movement of my legs with the rising stairs for a smooth pickup. Sadly, only my left leg coordinated well with its brain signal, whereas my right leg was a few nano-seconds behind. As Jennifer turned around to check on me, I was already at the beginning of an unwanted full leg split, and I am no gymnast! Spoiler alert: I somehow managed to stand up and continue our day.

At Jennifer's college graduation ceremony several years ago, I entered the coliseum lobby and accidentally separated from Abbey, Maura, and Sara within the crowd. As I looked for them, I happened upon a few very low steps and stopped to figure out how to conquer them without help and embarrassment. I stared at the small steps when, thankfully, a student representative with a big smile and huge heart gently took my arm, saying, "Let's do these together." Her kindness took the edge off my fears. The coliseum was constructed long before today's Americans with Disabilities Act requirements. Once inside the seating area, I faced many steep concrete stairs with no railings and narrow aisles awaiting my challenge. Abbey walked beside me, firmly gripping my arm, while Maura and Sara were in front, holding my hands as they bravely walked down backward. The stroke did not kill me, but surely these stairs would should I stumble. That is when I reminded them to save themselves should I stumble. "Don't worry about me. I still have eight more lives remaining," I shouted.

•• • ••

My nstagmus and disorientation toward spatial and perception relationships cause an inability to judge space or the straight-ahead position, "mid-line" as it is said accurately. Therefore, I tend to walk in a serpentine manner, zig-zagging, as I try to find the center point of my space. Serpentine walking, I joke, was an advantage for me while working in war zones overseas. My balance, posture, and ability to maintain a steady, rhythmic walking gait are difficult at best. Since the ground is a constant measure of spatial relationships, I keep my head down while walking, which is bad for proper posture. Most times, I fail to appreciate spatial cues on my right side, so I prefer someone who is walking beside me to be on my left side. Better still, I like to walk behind others so I am able to freely zig-zag.

After all, I still have eight more lives remaining

Chapter 3:
Navigating Life

I returned to work part-time within four and a half months post-stroke. Then I began working full-time shortly thereafter. The first day I returned to work, I walked to the meeting room with a few colleagues who had no idea of my deficits. I was flanked on all sides, so walking in a normal stride was impossible since I could not simultaneously digest numerous spatial relationship cues. I became too dizzy to understand where I was in space, so I moved to the outside perimeter of our pack, using the aisle wall as my constant reference point. Now, while being sandwiched between colleagues and the wall, I noticed a building facilities worker on a small ladder and painting the wall just ahead of us.

Even in my best controlled zigzag, I continually bumped into the wet wall, getting paint all over my suit's right sleeve and pant leg while trying to negotiate the aisle way. The painter was standing on the ladder, shaking his head, not believing his eyes. My colleagues laughed hysterically. I just said, "Damn stroke!" with a huge smirk on my face as the gang said, "Welcome back, Bryan!"

Survivors with Wallenberg's Syndrome sometimes report the world appears disturbingly tilted, making it difficult to maintain balance. This is very true for me as I have frequent bouts of unpleasant, near over-whelming dizziness, whereby I must stop all movements, rest, and re-settle myself for a few moments before resuming any activity.

The recovery rate for people with Wallenberg's symptoms depends on the area of the brain stem that the stroke has damaged; symptoms may decrease within weeks or months, or in my specific case, no appreciable decrease in nearly twenty years. However, some symptoms are now mitigated via-off-and-on therapy sessions and my learned ability to compensate when finding my new normal.

Maneuvering through crowds proves most challenging because I am trying to focus on people simultaneously coming toward me via several angles. I have difficulty processing all the visual information at a rate I can make sense of, and if I am not careful, disorientation and nausea may quickly take over. Crowd noises feel overly loud, thereby disrupting my concentration and interfering with my ability to pick up environmental cues. I do not like the sensation of feeling sandwiched or forced to walk normally when I cannot. When that happens, I move to the side, stand still, allow my environmental perception to settle down, and then resume walking.

However, when I stop walking, balancing myself in a standing position can prove problematic as the environment still feels as though it is moving. I react by taking, for example, Abbey's or my Girlies' hands to steady myself or look for an object to hold on to. On exercise walks, I steady myself by stopping and holding onto a tree branch, a bench, a pathway sign, or something else. If I have stopped to talk to a friend passing by and become dizzy as we converse, we simply laugh off my near-constant rocking motion. My friend may offer an arm to help steady me momentarily. However, if I have stopped for a passerby, momentarily holding that person is inappropriate or awkward, at the very least.

• • ● • •

To this very day, I wonder how I was able to lie perfectly still, feel safe, and obtain inner peace during the last brain scan attempt. My daughter, Maura, believes things happen in our lives for a reason that we later (or maybe not at all), realize and understand. Did the compassion of the technician who held my foot before I entered the tube calm me? Was it God's will? Perhaps my Uncle Solomon was looking after me from the spiritual world/afterlife? To help myself make some sense of what happened, I remember Uncle Solomon strongly believed in perspectives of having some sort of life after death; he often said, "There is something beyond the life we know, and God, or a representative of God, such as a family member, will be there for you in times of need."

Years after Uncle Solomon's death, but long before my stroke, I had a powerful dream, whereby I was with him again for a few moments. We were in the basement of my grandfather's general market, which I had never visited, yet the dream placed me there in some fabricated place in my mind. I was elated Uncle Solomon stood just a few feet away from me, and in his presence, I felt safe, peaceful, and blissful as if the world stood still. Speechless, I stared at the familiar attire he wore, smelled his favorite cologne, and then after a couple of seconds, in his strong baritone voice, he said, "We will never be able to do this again." I

While not outwardly religious, I hold God in my heart and mind. I believe God exists and am open to considering all viewpoints regarding God's existence and greatness. I have more questions than answers about God's role and will, especially now, as I continue trying to explain those defining moments inside the tube during the final attempt to obtain usable images. Though, I believe there must be a God because a couple of events in my life or in my family's life could not have been achieved without the miracle of a supreme being!

suspect this meant we would never see each other again in the world as I understand it to be.

Extending my arm, I reached out to him just as he disappeared.

- Was this a powerful dream, or did it really happen?
- Was this Uncle Solomon's way of showing me there is indeed another life after death?
- Was Uncle Solomon with me as God's representative, confirming a family member would be there for us in our times of need?

I had entered the tube for what I believed would be my last chance to survive if the technicians were not able to obtain useful brain scan images?

...in his presence, I felt safe, peaceful, and blissful as if the world stood still.

CHAPTER 4:
ABBEY

On the day of my stroke, Abbey and Eldon arrived at the second hospital later that afternoon. Then, my brother, Alan, arrived. Seeing them reinforced my feelings of being comforted and safe. Abbey's reassuring expression and holding my hand reminded me I would be fine moving forward. Exhausted from the day's training run and a flurry of tests, I have little memory of their visit. I just wanted to hold Abbey's hand and fall asleep. However, the doctor politely reiterated that I could not sleep until all the tests were evaluated. Then, Abbey and Eldon spoke to the doctor privately about what happened and the next steps of care. Eldon and Alan began playing their big brother roles, keeping the mood upbeat. Alan wished he could do more to help me, and the two of them looked out for Abbey. She is strong, calm, cool, and collected while handling unnerving situations with a positive *let's just take care of this* mentality.

Since the day I met Abbey, she has proven strong, compassionate, and independent. Of all her positive qualities as a spouse, best friend, mother, and hard worker in and outside the home, these character traits absolutely stand out. Our family can always count on Abbey for strength, positive thoughts, and hopes.

Several years after my stroke, Abbey was diagnosed with advanced stage three breast cancer. Her strength and constant optimism from the beginning never wavered, making her recovery look easy! She faced each day head-on with that same *let's just take care of this* mentality and move forward bit by bit with a positive attitude, while ensuring our family was cared for. I was absolutely in awe of her courage and how she took charge of her recovery.

Abbey received excellent care and assistance from our Girlies, family, friends, and medical teams. I am convinced Abbey's unwavering positivity significantly influenced her speedy recovery. Abbey is an example of strength for all of us to admire and follow. She is an absolutely fantastic role model for our daughters, friends, and other family members, and I see these same strong qualities in my Girlies. They have endured my stroke, Abbey's breast cancer, and their own personal hardships at such very young ages, yet they moved very successfully forward in life with their own powerful strength and resolve! I am so very proud of them! My family is a constant role model for me!

Abbey and I did not need life-altering events to put life's perspective back in order. We already fully recognized how fortunate we were and how precious life is every time we see our three wonderful, successful, *down-to-earth* daughters.

My family is a constant role model for me!

Chapter 5: Rehabilitation

When my stroke ended later that evening, my case was studied and reports written after all the scans, imaging, and tests were evaluated. Doctors and specialists made a final diagnosis and assessment of how much brain damage had occurred so they could develop what care needs would look like presently and in the longer term. Many stroke specialists now believe it is critical to participate in early, diligent rehabilitation therapy exercises as soon as possible in hopes of mitigating or reversing as much stroke damage as possible.

Early rehabilitation is believed to assist recovery efforts, hopefully at a faster rate of time and allow a survivor to potentially have the best meaningful recovery chances. In many cases, survivors obtain the most significant recovery during the first three to six months after a stroke. However, please note that today's re-

During phase two, neurons actively grow new connections called synapses. As these neurons build new synapses, they change how they communicate with one another. Communication gets stronger between some neurons, while other lines of communication weaken, a give and take [process], allowing the brain to adapt to an injury. The injured brain also makes another adjustment by engaging new areas of the brain to do the job [that other neurons completed] or [re-engaging the] injured area. When phase two ends, the brain gets harder to work with.

search proves recovery remains possible even multiple years later. Neurologists are now saying there is no timetable to continue improving, even from a severe stroke, regardless of time. Whether these improvements are in basic movements, motor skills, reasoning, and on and on, a survivor has the ability to make gains at any point. I am proof of ongoing positive gains even though I am nearly twenty years post-stroke. Never give up hope! Keep a positive attitude! And understand stroke recovery can be lengthy! So do not become discouraged!

In spring of 2012, Dr. Steven C. Cramer, professor of neurology, anatomy, and neurobiology at the University of California, Irvine, reported in *Stroke Connection* magazine that recovery from a stroke is divided into three distinct phases.

> **Phase One:** Doctors try to limit injury caused by a stroke at the time it is taking place. He states that within hours of a stroke, the brain goes into a repair mode.

> **Phase Two:** The brain undergoes a growth spurt; it is during this phase the brain is receptive to reformatting.

> **Phase Three:** The brain becomes less able to reconfigure. There is still potential for change but not as great as the potential in the second phase.

It is during this phase that survivors may become frustrated as their hopeful progress perhaps has slowed down at a critical point of their therapy progression, delaying continued advancement.

I was well observed and cared for until the wee hours of the morning while in the emergency room and then moved to Intensive Care (IC). I joked with the transporters as they wheeled me to IC about pulling a few wheelies just so part of this long day could at least be fun. Once in IC, I was allowed to sleep for a few hours.

I was momentarily confused when I woke up and tried to figure out where I was and what would happen next. I quickly noticed simple sounds irritated me, such as the loud conversations within the hallway, the soft sounds from the heart monitor, the blood pressure monitor, and even the hum of the compression machine for the packs on my legs. I did not think too much about any *slight* annoyance at the time, but it later became a precursor to one of my irrational behaviors: anger. The American Stroke Association states, "After a stroke or brain injury, a survivor may become highly sensitive to sound." Stroke can affect the auditory processing areas of the brain, causing heightened sensitivity to sounds even at low volumes. This is a common side effect and termed auditory overload (AO). Your brain feels as though you are receiving too much sensory stimuli and has a difficult time processing the information.

While living at the hospitals, noise and sound sensitivities were not as evident, seemingly having little effect on me. Perhaps, I had a better tolerance level because I was not usually over-stimulated and so tired. Once discharged and back in normal environments, I became decidedly susceptible to certain sounds and pitches, such as the slamming shut of any door, drawer, cabinet, or higher pitched sounds/screams, whether a voice, machine, or loud engine. Even the clanging of pots, pans, and dishes are just a few noises that bother me. These sounds raise my frustration level, which, in turn, becomes upsetting, and there is nothing I can do about it except wear earplugs. My interpretation of noise remains an issue today because I feel nearly constantly as though my ears hurt or my brain feels exhausted. I have earplugs readily available for those *just in case moments*. If I am attending a private social event, I do not want to inadvertently insult the host. So, I casually mention why I am wearing them and assure the host that everything is fine.

In the summer of 2013, Mr. Jon Caswell wrote an article for *Stroke Connection* magazine. The title of the article was "Sound Advice." This article stated that "Survivors with Auditory Overload may become more isolated because they are reluctant to go into challenging social environments and instead stay home."

I have politely passed on opportunities to go out because of concerns regarding noise depending upon the venue. Luckily, friends and family appreciate my concern and allow me to bow out gracefully. Otherwise, if appropriate, I ask people if they would mind changing the meeting venue. If friends wanted to go to a popular bar and grill, I might suggest another place that is equally acceptable but perhaps not as loud or busy.

While in IC, a stroke expert/specialist and his team took over my care, calling for additional frequent brain scans, which meant several gurney rides to the scanning room. On one occasion, we arrived to find the room was in use. The transporters were instructed to leave me in the hallway because a technician would receive me momentarily. Alone in the hallway, I was a bit scared before a technician, doctor, nurse, or staff member came out of the room. In my slight voice, I called out telling her I had a stroke only hours ago and remained nervous, a tad bit anxious, and just did not want to be alone. She was compassionate and reassuring during our short conversation before going back inside the scanning room. Moments later, I was moved into the room for my scans. Then I was wheeled back to IC and told to rest before neurologists would revisit me soon.

Over the next few days, I had multiple tubes inserted into my nose, one of which was a feeding tube, a Nasogastric Tube (NG), that carries food and medicine to the stomach through the nose because I had and still have a severely weakened muscular ability to swallow anything including my saliva. I used a suction tube to clear out the saliva that would build up in my mouth for the first several weeks of my hospital stay. Today, swallowing remains problematic, but I am far better at managing food and liquid, only choking a couple of times a week versus every day.

Abbey and I were at our daughter Sara's residence, watching a movie and eating popcorn when I suddenly began choking. I quickly sat up from my chair and hurriedly tried walking to the kitchen sink to spit out the contents in my mouth. I did not make it too far before passing out for maybe three seconds from not being able to breathe correctly. While going down, I set off a chain reaction, culminating in knocking over Sara's bicycle, causing damage and complete embarrassment. Note to self: scratch popcorn from my list of things to eat! Sometimes, trial and error teach me what I can or cannot eat. I have had several modified barium swallow studies for food and liquids and the chances for aspiration pneumonia. I try my best not to eat in front of anyone, including family and friends, or at least mitigate these opportunities as much as possible for fear of choking in front of them and causing a scene. Admittedly, I sometimes *shoot myself in the foot* by eating faster than I should—an old habit. I was the runt of my parent's litter; having three older brothers forced me to eat fast and fend for myself at the dinner table.

· · ● · ·

Each morning the hospital physical therapist visited me to assess my abilities to move my body, be it arms, legs, neck, head, or core area. She was pleasantly surprised I wanted these daily therapies, saying patients usually want to remain in bed a little longer, but I was happy for the light exercise and to prove I would return to my *normal,* hopefully, quickly. Plus, I was very excited to go to Alaska, now departing in three days. Unfortunately, I had tunnel vision, fixated on leaving the hospital quickly by proving I was well enough to do all things planned as scheduled. When Abbey and the neurologists told me the severity of my stroke and that traveling to Alaska was not an option, I could not accept the news. I was distraught, heartbroken, and disillusioned all at once, overwhelmed by thoughts of *now what?* What, if anything, will be *normal again?*

I had little time to *drown in my sorrow.* Since I could not swallow properly, doctors ordered a more involved procedure called a stomach gastrostomy to ensure proper nutritional levels were maintained. A small surgical incision was made to place a feeding tube directly into my stomach. Ironically, during the gastrostomy procedure, the charge doctor was the very same person who helped calm me while waiting alone outside the scanning room. I did not recognize her at first, but I was comforted knowing she would oversee the procedure because it felt like another friend cared for me. I used this feeding tube for multiple months until learning to swallow safely without choking or aspirating.

After a couple of weeks at the second hospital, my condition was stabilized and my neurologist felt it was now best to transport me to a live-in rehabilitation hospital with an intensive, specialty stroke facility for daily in-depth rehabilitation care in physical, cognitive, occupational, speech and activities of daily living (ADL) therapies. (For more information, go to the Appendix.) I absolutely received the best level of care, compassion, and truly amazing lifesaving medical attention at the two initial hospitals. I am so very fortunate to be alive because of the staffs at both hospitals.

I will forever credit them for their heroic actions.

CHAPTER 6:
THE THIRD HOSPITAL

N ow, infirmed at the third hospital, I had other heroes who continued professional, compassionate care. The first day was everything administrative: settling in. Abbey and I met the unit managing nurse. She made it politely clear that I am here to work, and they would push me to work, if necessary. I told her that was perfectly fine, stating, "I respond best in a strong, structured environment. Count on me to work hard at recovering. Just give me the tools to help myself!"

I would be their patient for a long time, so Abbey was thrust into playing multiple roles simultaneously as a spouse, caregiver, mom, dual parent, emotional support provider for all of us, and coordinator of all things for the kids. Whether it was their school activities, multiple sports activities, practices, games, going to appointments, their healthcare needs, carpools, social events, extracurricular activities, meals, cleaning, and giving time to our family dog, Abbey had no time for herself. Simply visiting me was a two-hour round-trip drive, not including visitation time. Very little time was available for Abbey to accomplish to-do lists or even unwind for her well-being. Abbey very humbly fulfilled these responsibilities, saying, "There was not a day that went by that I was not exhausted and overwhelmed, yet I carried on. I had to be strong and give our family the best care possible." What an amazingly strong person!

At this hospital, I had to prove I could care for myself before eventually returning home. My first few days of in-depth physical, occupational, cognitive, speech, ADL, and periodic mental health therapies were faced with humbling circumstances as I now focused full-time strictly on rehabilitation. I began completing physical therapies immediately, genuinely enjoying the sessions because they were a powerful physical and mental healing process and motivator. Each day, I had a mixture of ALL therapies with an initial focus on exercising and stimulating my throat muscles in hopes of increasing my capability to swallow normally and get a variety of food nutrients and calories to stabilize my rapid weight loss from solely being fed liquid nutrients via a tube, often referred to as a G-tube. These swallowing therapies included electro-stimulation, which forced my throat muscles to move in hopes of initiating stronger muscle movements and control so I could return to regular food consumption To stimulate muscle movement, probes were attached to my neck to produce muscle contractions and squeezes. It was not hurtful; in fact, there was an upside to this therapy. I was chewing and attempting to swallow food while being closely observed. This therapy provided an indulgent taste of comfort food and its flavors. In my first session with the therapist, I was instructed to consume a tiny amount of crunchy candy and light thin chips. Depending on how I reacted, the therapist slowly introduced applesauce and other foods. I was self-conscious of her observing and listening to my throat muscles respond as I chewed with hopeful expectations of swallowing properly soon. Day one provided a baseline measurement of my muscles' abilities, which were less optimistic than anyone desired. I did not care about the findings in some ways because they were just a starting point for providing the therapists with valuable data for developing a therapeutic program. Besides, I was in nirvana trying to eat comfort food. When swallowing became problematic, exercises were stopped, but the chewing mechanics continued, allowing the therapist to observe how I managed the contents in my mouth before eventually spitting out the food. I savored the flavors without the calories. It was empty, mindless enjoyment! So mindless, while practicing swallowing therapies, I chewed my way through an eighteen-ounce bag of milk chocolate candy—the different colored ones with the hard shells.

Unfortunately, my swallowing abilities were the last muscle group to produce any improvement, so I had to continue relying on tube feeding myself for multiple months. As more and more time passed with little to no improvement, I viewed tube feeding as a chore versus the pleasantries of a normal meal or snack. I especially became dejected when Abbey would make her delicious family meals, with all the splendor of tasty aromas, and I could not partake. I eventually lost thirty-three pounds in eight weeks. My assigned nutritionist and others provided a concerned warning that my body will not be able to keep up with the demands of rehabilitation therapies if I do not *feed* myself properly, and any gains I have made to this point might suffer a setback. Well, that is all the motivation I needed to get back on track of tube feeding at consistent intervals. I cannot explain it, but being hungry while tube feeding was for me very, very different than being hungry because I had not eaten food in a while. I could go hours upon hours between tube feedings, but when eating food, if I did not eat at proper intervals, I often had headaches or became *hangry*: a slang word using a combination of the words hungry and angry.

Abbey visited me every day. I could be myself around her, joke around, complete my exercises in front of her, cry, and feel sorry for myself for an occasional moment. I did not share my fears and burdens during hers or family visits, especially not when my Girlies visited. Their *job* was to be normal kids as much as possible, not worrying about their father or other *adult things*. Though I wanted to calmly explain my stroke and tell them I would be home soon, I did not know if I could answer their potential questions or provide the right balance of information given their young ages. I feared overwhelming them or, worse, compromising their coping mechanisms. I tried to protect them from our reality, but that only confused them about what was happening—not just to me, but rightfully and most importantly, what was happening in their world, which SUDDENLY changed. My stroke did not just affect me. It affected and shocked my family as we confronted our new reality, and Abbey was now solely juggling the family needs, work, and the demands of caregiving full-time.

I needed more time to appropriately sort through all the thoughts racing inside my head before talking to my Girlies. However, delaying meant they had less understanding of the bigger picture, so they naturally gravitated to Abbey for answers and nearly everything else as I grew more and more angry and insecure. I read an article written by Jon Caswell in *Stroke Connection* magazine dated September/October 2010. In the article, he stated, "Children may have great frustration and confusion as they try to navigate a relationship that may have changed dramatically." In addition, Caswell noted younger survivors between twenty and fifty have challenges that older survivors may not face, chiefly the concerns of raising children after stroke, reactions from other people, loss of friends, and loss of a career. These were my fears too. I completely empathized with Mr. Caswell's article. My fears and insecurities were mine alone. I could not burden my family with them.

> So, I went about my days with a quiet *move forward* in recovery—*fix problems later.* Recovery was for better or worse my priority one.

Every morning, I woke up early and readied myself for therapy, excited to begin feeling productive via exercise. As much as was possible, my mindset was I would do everything I could do for myself. I considered everything I did a therapy of some sort. My routine became brushing my teeth, sometimes my chin or nose, because of weakened hand/eye coordination. I attempted a cursory sponge bath followed by dressing myself. Usually, it took me forty-five minutes to put on a shirt, tidy whities, socks, shorts, and brush my hair, while also navigating my wheelchair. It did not matter how long my routine too or if I struggled a bit because maybe, just maybe, the next day I would be faster at getting ready for the day using less effort. I ABSOLUTELY had to know I tried and that I did everything possible to help myself heal. Then and only then, I'd ask for God's help. If I never healed, then so be it. Somehow, I would have to learn how to cope with the fate imparted upon me. Here, too, I would need God's help. But I would have peace knowing I gave everything I could of myself to heal. When I finished my morning routine, the rehabilitation specialist would come by to let me know the day's game plan. Each day, I accomplished tiny improvements, which helped me maintain an optimistic outlook and feel less of a burden, less scared, and more invigorated for the next challenge. I fully believed I would make greater strides soon or somehow gain the courage to adjust to this life-altering event. Even on the days I struggled, several rehabilitation therapists were impressed by my determination to continue working on the day's program. Admittedly, always believing in myself was ambitious. Patience is not a strong virtue of mine, but feeling sorry for myself certainly was not an option nor was being reticent to take my first steps, pun intended, toward a successful outcome.

These accomplishments fueled a stronger mental stamina, allowing me to set my sights beyond what was in front of me. To keep progressing, I had to allow myself to have complete faith in others and ask and accept the graciousness of their assistance. The most challenging part for me was learning patience. But, more than anything, I desired God's assistance in helping Abbey and my Girlies through their most difficult days. I was not sure I deserved God's help. I did not always know what struggles they were experiencing. Abbey wanted me to concentrate on my healing and not worry about them, so she only shared the easier parts of their day, and I was so focused on my situation, I didn't ask the tougher questions.

After therapy sessions, I had many hours of free time with few distractions. I was unable to read or watch television because of my poor quality of vision, and I did not want anyone other than Abbey visiting because I was self-conscious about my thin, fragile appearance and feeling less than a viable man. Looking at myself in the mirror was worrisome enough. I did not want others to see me this way. Abbey wanted to bring the kids during her visits, but I requested she not do so, thinking I was protecting them and ensuring they did not miss anopportunity to be playful and enjoy their day however they desired. Of course, they had homework and chores to complete! In hindsight, frequent family visits could have been inclusive time toward helping us heal and feeling better together.

Boredom and over-thinking quickly became my enemy at the end of the day, allowing my mind to swirl with worries. I had to *keep it together.* To remain encouraged, I visualized cheerful moments of wonderful family togetherness. A mental health doctor reinforced what I read many years earlier about the benefits of using positive visualization as a powerful tool to help heal and achieve desires.

We discussed the scientific proof of how visualization helps create a mind-body connection to strengthen a person's well-being and why this fact is taught to young children combating adverse health circumstances. I envisioned walking again without help, exercising, riding bikes with the kids, getting back to participating in their sports activities, enjoying more wonderful family vacations, and having beautiful thoughts of going back home surrounded by Abbey and my *Girlies, and on and on.*

I also thought about how my Uncle Solomon would find some possible good from something awful. Despite my life-altering event, I had hoped to show that I was not caught up in self-pity and *why me* attitudes. I wanted to be an example for my family to draw strength from by proving I was recovering well and remaining capable of doing things as I did before my stroke. I was determined not to let the stroke compare and contrast me as the Bryan before stroke and the Bryan after stroke. It would simply be a blip on the screen. Sadly, I lost sight of my goals without the structured setting of the hospitals once I returned home. So, things indeed became noticeably changed. Though I was recovering remarkably well, given my circumstances, it was not fast enough for me.

I was not the person I envisioned post-stroke.

CHAPTER 7:
ACTIVITIES OF DAILY
LIVING (ADL)

My first **activity of daily living** (ADL) therapy was an actual shower for the first time in several weeks rather than a sponge bath. A simple shower was going to *make my day!* One embarrassing concern: my therapist was a young woman who would teach me how to shower safely alone, dress myself, and become more attentive to my surroundings. That day's ADL lesson began with learning how to transfer from my wheelchair to the shower bench. I wore all my clothes, and she asked, "Have you always taken a shower with clothes on?"

Slightly embarrassed, I replied, "I did not know I was taking an actual shower now. I thought I was just going to demonstrate my ability to transfer from the wheelchair to the shower bench (albeit not so gracefully), and then be alone in the bathroom to shower."

She handed me a towel, closed the shower curtain, and said, "For your safety, I must be in the bathroom." I was reticent to undress behind the curtain, then shower, and come out with just a towel on. Knowing I was embarrassed, she said, "No worries. I have assisted many patients, and you will be covered up by your towel."

To which I replied, "I understand that, but you have not assisted me before. Besides, didn't you say you are getting married shortly?"

"Why does that matter?" she asked.

I jokingly replied, "Because seeing me wearing just a towel might make you rethink getting married as I am no longer in strong physical shape."

•••●•••

The hospital had a mock apartment setup within the therapy area for home ADL practice. The staff required me to demonstrate abilities to work and maneuver within the confines of varying rooms using my wheelchair, walker, quad cane, and regular cane to make a bed, vacuum, clean, and cook. A therapist asked if I would make my specialty meatloaf for the staff. I talked about family dinners and how I missed them. Making a meal at the hospital would serve two purposes. I would be able to demonstrate my capabilities to work within the kitchen and offer enjoyment as we socialized sharing a meal together. It served a third purpose. I truly missed family dinner time with my Girlies and Abbey; this opportunity allowed me to feel I was in a family environment.

At home, my Girlies were ever so thankful Abbey made us dinners, but now and then they let me try to make a meal, usually a simple meatloaf and a chicken loaf for Sara, served with homemade mashed potatoes and veggies. My dinners barely qualified as a meal, but my Girlies seemed to enjoy them. Although, more than likely, they had excellent game faces! I have very fond memories of making the meals and teaching them how I made the loaves.

That day's meal ADL was indeed practical, and I felt comforted surrounded by staff, eating together as a mock family. Happily, no one became sick. However, I accidentally discovered I could touch HOT pans/dishes without feeling the heat sensation. I knew the left side of my body had weakened muscles and diminished feelings in my arm, leg, and foot. However, until this incident, I did not recognize that the right side of my body did not feel temperature and had diminished sensations.

·•●•·

Fast forward a few months. Abbey went out with friends for the evening and asked my brother, Eldon, to babysit me. I made us meatloaf for dinner and decided to play a joke on him by reaching my right hand into the oven without wearing a potholder to fetch the loaf pan. The look on Eldon's face was priceless. After my hardy laugh, he told me that I may not feel the extreme heat, but I could severely burn my skin. Well, so much for my hardy laugh! I don't do things like that anymore. However, I enter pools, lakes, or oceans, dipping the right side of my body first. This condition also mitigates the winter cold or summer heat feel on that side of my body. In addition, I don't have to purchase jackets with a right-arm sleeve, so I save a bit of money.

·•●•·

After weeks of using a pee bottle or calling for assistance to use the toilet, I developed greater therapeutic motivation to learn how to transfer out of the hospital bed into the wheelchair alone against all hospital protocols. I would make my way to the bathroom, then transfer out of the wheelchair to the toilet, then reverse everything. The entire process wasn't pretty or skilled, but I would marvel at my accomplishment. Being cleaned with assistance was immensely embarrassing, and while I recognize embarrassment should not be a concern in most all circumstances, I was self-conscious about this unwanted attention. While entirely grateful for the assistance, I wanted to take over that ADL action. Hospital staff would tell me with polite anger to please use the Call Button and ask for help rather than try to do things independently. I would playfully tell them I would next find a way to stand while I pee, and a nurse asked with a smile, "What is it with men wanting to stand? All my male patients want to stand; what's the big deal? You guys drive me crazy with your nonsense!"

•●●●•

The staff personnel at each hospital played vital roles to ensure I achieved the best possible recovery outcome. I will always remain grateful for their care, genuine concern, compassion, skill, and expertise, which gave me the best chance to survive, recover, and go home amazingly functional.

After two months of rigorous therapies and solid gains, I was discharged.

CHAPTER 8:
WORRIES

While I was proud of working diligently at becoming independent again, I would now be away from expert rehabilitation specialists who provided structured care, an accepting environment, and the necessary encouragement to get my life back together. I was extremely apprehensive about leaving a protected, controlled hospital cocoon. I quickly found comfort in placing all my trust in them during the most difficult health challenge of my life. They helped me navigate and cope with the *uncharted waters* post-stroke and helped me manage the ups and downs of recovering while cheering on my determination to heal. I had been solely focused on recovering via physical, cognitive, and speech therapies and regaining the ability to perform all ADLs while living in a relatively quiet atmosphere with limited outside environmental stimuli and distractions. I was not yet in a *real-world setting,* so it was easier to maintain a laser focus on healing. I was scared about leaving the hospital. Once home, though nervous, I was so happy to be home and surrounded by my Girlies and Abbey!

Abbey prepared the house exceptionally well for my safe and comfortable transition home. Moments before I entered the house, I faced the first home challenge of my disability: the two steps up to the porch leading to the front door. I smiled at the irony, but Abbey devised a quick solution.

She wheeled me into the garage where there was only one smaller step to negotiate and muscled me inside the house while I remained seated in my wheelchair.

Instead of relishing the moment of finally being home, I looked around the house, quickly worrying about Abbey and me potentially losing what we built for our family, ourselves, and careers. Would we be able to pay the mortgage and stay in our neighborhood? Living modestly, should I not be able to return to work and remain an equal provider? How do Abbey and I tell our daughters their lives must change because mine changed? Yes, we would adjust, but that was not what was going through my mind at that moment in time. I could not bear to burden my family or possibly alter their lifestyle.

I cried over unrelenting worries about my capability to remain a viable, equal provider, supporter, husband, father, and man. I was a lost soul, ashamed of my stroke and now ashamed of my evolving *ugly, angry, new self* and frightened of losing my family's need of me. I obsessed nearly daily about my family's welfare, health, and emotional well-being. Yet, ironically, it was me causing so much damage. I worried about my ability to recover and regain control of my impulsive, angry behaviors. I was not in a woe-is-me or self-pity mindset. These are normal concerns and questions for anyone having had a life-altering event. My feelings were not unique.

In a report from John Hopkins Hospital, Generalized Anxiety Disorder (GAD) was the subject. GAD is characterized as a tendency to worry a lot about everyday issues and situations. The worry is constant without the ability to control it.

On my first night home, I woke Abbey in the wee hours of the morning, needing assistance to get to the bathroom just thirteen feet from my bedside. I was still learning to walk and was unstable even using my walker. Having Abbey walk alongside me, reassured me I would not go *ten toes up*. It took me several minutes to get out of bed and cover the short distance. I nearly peed myself twice! While most would be discouraged, I was proud of myself. I reached the bathroom toilet, so I considered it a victory!

Home life tested every aspect of my deficits, known and not yet realized. These pertained to the physical, hearing, emotional, and even intimacy. I went from a decent, caring person straight to ugly anger, bypassing all the normal steps of coping with grief. I had no coping skills or mechanisms in place to face this challenge. I relied heavily upon being able to own my recovery under my terms and return to being a nice guy. Caring people in my world would say warmhearted things: "Go easy on yourself." "Take things one day at a time." "The best is yet to come." All of their comments were well- intended, but I needed tangible, actionable skills.

Abbey suggested making a temporary bedroom for me on the middle level to avoid stairs, but I wanted to be with family as much as possible. I used my wheelchair on the middle level, then went upstairs on my tush, using the banister for lifting and pulling. I became decently proficient at this method and would proudly smirk as I reminded Abbey or my Girlies where my documents were should I wipe out. Other times, I would hold onto someone with one arm and white knuckle grip the banister with the other arm while moving my legs slowly and deliberately as we climbed each stair together. Usually, mid-way, I asked if anyone needed a rest, snack, or drink—trying to be funny. Once safely upstairs, I used my walker or cane to help move around.

Though I said from the beginning of my recovery journey that life happens, and all I needed was the knowledge and tools to heal. Regretfully, I had no fathomable idea I was facing a *new me*, my hidden disability. I did not understand my brain had changed. I simply thought I would return home as my normal self with a few necessary mobility changes but easily continuing everyday family life. There were no mental health discussions or therapies on potential personality changes during my rehabilitation stays. Hindsight has been an enemy to this day. It can be a great teacher or, in my case, a regretful reminder if only I had understood *this* or *done that* instead. My family and I were totally unprepared for my personality and behavior changes. During this awful time, my family endured my horrible temperament while trying to balance their own life needs, emotions, understanding, and health.

More than at any other time, I needed my family, yet my behavior rightfully discouraged them from wanting to be with me. Any form of intimacy between Abbey and me quickly diminished and then ended. Simply holding hands was not an option. Then, as Abbey wanted less and less to do with me, I retaliated with more anger—a terrible spiraling circumstance. Any marital concerns I had prior to my stroke, I now aired out as I was no longer bashful to state what was on my mind. Unfortunately, most comments were unfiltered and, therefore, not constructive.

I retaliated with more anger—a terrible spiraling circumstance.

CHAPTER 9:
ADLs AT HOME

I had difficulty functioning in a typical home environment. I was frustrated as I tried to work through everyday life events. I struggled to keep pace with the normal flow of activities, and create order *when I could not sort the pile.* Home life now seemed like a hustle and bustle of things to accomplish not the order and structure I had grown accustomed to. Compounding my efforts to face the *real world,* was my frequent mental, physical, medication, and stroke fatigue over stimulation. This fatigue had nothing at all to do with quality sleep or any sleeping issue. It was solely my mind and body were tired from the stroke effects. Sometimes, I felt taxed from the day's events and needed rest, so I would withdraw to a quiet area, hoping to manage the stimuli before becoming overwhelmed and agitated. Leaving eliminated the possibility of projecting my anger, frustrations, and insecurity onto my family. However, leaving came with unintended consequences of being seen as a husband and dad who does not want to participate in any family activity, only caring about himself.

I struggled to adjust back to everyday life and routines. I became frustrated and angry at benign *things* for no justifiable reason. This *new me* was ugly, and no amount of guidance or *heads-up* could have adequately braced my family for my misguided negative behavior, emotional needs, or *wild* anxieties that often unproductively surfaced. The only consistent, sure feelings I had were for the happiness I wished for my wife and Girlies and wanting to see their usual smiles and zest in their hearts. This sentiment will always hold true! I wish this type of behavior exhibited itself rather than anger!

It was much easier to manage and accept the compensations I must make in the cognitive, physical, speech, and ADL challenges than the damage I inflicted on my family and the guilt I will forever carry within me as I fought to defeat my *new me*. I make no excuses, fully owning up to my negative behaviors. I will be forever scarred by my verbal anger toward my family. Through everything we experienced together, my wife Abbey and my Girlies remained by my side with a rightful degree of guarded hope. I maintained a cautious belief in myself when others were unsure.

Chapter 10:
No Way Around Ugliness

I sincerely made peace with what fate had imparted upon me soon after my stroke. I simply desired to work at moving forward with renewed perspectives of life's precious time and its wonders. I remained a lucky man and never thought otherwise! I still had what truly matters: family, friends, our bonding connections, and love. My mind and heart told God how grateful I was to have survived, but I did not act appreciative. I wanted to be helpful and productive at home, rather than a burden, but I was consumed with trying to comprehend how the very being of who I was changed beyond my control. I did not recognize myself; I hated this *new me*!

I was selfish, had unprovoked anger fits, and bouts of please-understand-what I-am-going-through. I foolishly believed my family would unquestionably accept what was happening to us and did not initially consider they were truly hurting as well as I tried to make sense of everything. My Girlies only saw a small piece of the puzzle. They deserved an explanation of what was happening although I believed this was all temporary, and I would soon return to *my normal self.* I completely underestimated the power of the brain, which was the nexus for almost all my mistakes post-stroke.

However, I was wholly unprepared to understand that a powerful, ugly *new me* had evolved, which turned our lives upside down. I used to keep my emotions rational and *in check*. Now, I was all over the place with how I felt and then asking myself if my feelings are justified. I remain feeling guilty for becoming sick during the most impressionable and vital time of my Girlies' lives and for not being a role model. I do not blame my stroke for the pain I caused my family. I will always take unconditional responsibility and hold myself accountable for hurting Abbey and my Girlies.

According to The Stroke Foundation, a condition called *emotional liability* is common after a stroke.

> This is when emotional responses don't seem to make much sense or are out of proportion; your emotional responses may appear out of character or be out of context.

> This is also known as the Pseudobulbar Affect. Survivors may strongly react intensely to the most minor thing upsetting them.

It also states, "Sometimes, changes in behavior are aimed only at the people closest to the stroke survivor. This is quite normal."

> Most of us only show the more difficult parts of ourselves to the people we are closest to because we know they will probably forgive us. However, if the behavior is extreme, it can isolate us from the people around us. Sometimes, stroke survivors do not realize their behaviors or personalities are different. This can make it difficult to address these changes. Existing personality traits may become more pronounced, or people may behave in ways that are out of character. After a stroke, it can feel like you are no longer the same person you were before. Stroke survivors, partners (spouses), and family members can all feel grief about

this. Everybody needs to find their way of coping with these changes and this will take time.

My family will attest to my irrational responses. For example, a few weeks after being discharged, I asked my Girlies to please clean their rooms before going out for the day. They begrudgingly began. Then, when finished, I started my inspection. No Girlie passed my inspection because of simple fuzz on the floor, or clothes were not hung up or placed in a dresser drawer. Pre-stroke me would have simply asked them to complete touch-ups of a couple of areas of their room, then I'd leave. Post-stroke me actually yelled at them and carried on for not doing things to my liking. My response was not at all proportionate to the task at hand.

I pride myself on being clean, organized, and completing tasks purposefully and on time. This purposeful driven character trait is just who I am, but now that side of me became exasperated sometimes upsetting Abbey as I become frustrated after vacuuming the floors of dog hair only to discover something else got on the floor. Since retiring, I am more of a moderate Type A personality, predominantly Type B personality.

It is important to know that someone who appears outwardly healthy can still have a disability often termed an *invisible wound*. Many therapists and others in the medical profession use this term to describe, for example, a returning soldier with no outwardly apparent injury. Yet, she or he may have suffered a brain injury.

The Airforce Wounded Warrior Program states,

> An invisible wound is a cognitive, emotional, or behavioral condition that can be associated with trauma or serious adverse life events. Examples of possible diagnoses are major depressive disorder, post-traumatic stress disorder, PTSD, and traumatic brain injury, TBI."

Those having a stroke or another type of brain injury, I believe, suffer from an invisible wound as well.

My brain trauma may not be readily apparent, but I am a changed person.

· • ● • ·

According to AARP author Oliver Broudy, in an article he entitled "When Seconds Count," he writes, "Strokes are among the most feared medical emergencies. What else but a stroke could make you think you'd rather have a heart attack? Sure, heart attacks are more fatal, but at least if you survive, you can carry on more or less as before without a dimming of the mind or loss of key bodily functions." Broudy also writes in the same article, Time is ESSENTIAL, minutes matter [there is only] a short window of time in which the devastating effects of a stroke could perhaps be mitigated. It is reported only 1.3 percent of people receive treatment in the first hour [of their stroke] and nearly twenty percent are treated between three and four and a half hours after its onset. For every thirty-minute delay, the relative likelihood of surviving a stroke with no deficits decreases by fifteen percent.

> During an overseas assignment, Abbey informed me I became a victim of identity theft. Thieves somehow learned of my credit card number and used it to purchase whatever they wanted. Upon learning I was a victim, I filled out the customary merchant and police reports with notations stating I did not even want to be me, so why would someone else want to be me?

My cognitive functions immediately post-stroke were fine, thank goodness! I realized I had periodic brain hiccups when feeling *overloaded*, so putting two and two together was sometimes delayed. Thank goodness again, everything quickly returned to normal within weeks of my stroke. Now, I tell people teaching me something once would be okay. Quite frankly, you are better off teaching me twice, and stay on standby because you might have to reach out a third time.

These brain hiccups continue, so I must pay close attention and actively listen. Just ask Abbey, LOL! I write myself reminder notes in the old-fashioned manner of using a scrap piece of paper. There are no devices to log onto, no passwords to remember, and no power failures. I only need a pant pocket or counter top for my note to rest in/on.

Keeping pace with fast or multiple simultaneous conversations is tricky because while the person speaking may be on sentence nine, I might be lagging and processing sentence six. Sometimes when conversing with someone, words or thoughts may get stuck on the other side of my brain where a pathway has been affected, so it may take me a couple seconds to process and convey my intent. Please don't finish my thought or rush me to say something. If I am genuinely stuck expressing myself, a gentle push is welcomed. Otherwise, please let me speak. Sit back, smoke a stogie, or drink a beer while giving me an extra moment to process my thoughts. An interruption may cause me to completely lose everything. In an interview with another survivor, JW, he said, "I gotta finish a thought uninterrupted; don't finish my sentence even if you know what I am going to say because sometimes I just need to finish for myself, so I can sequence the next thought."

Not long after I returned home, Abbey arranged a neighborhood guys-only night out so I could celebrate with friends after being cooped up for several months. I suspect she just wanted me out of the house, allowing her a chance to breathe! As I put on my jacket that evening, I stared at it, realizing I wasn't sure what to do first. I went in with both arms first so it appeared as if I were wearing a straight jacket. I panicked; something was oddly wrong. To save face, I laughed heartedly as if I were doing sight gags on a comedy show. Abbey subtly assisted me with an, "Oh Bryan, silly boy," blowing it off as comedy too. I believe the guys did not think anything of it—at least not openly.

I was putting groceries in the refrigerator while holding my wallet and keys. They were in my right hand, and I struggled to grab and grip a carton of orange juice in my post-stroke, weaker left hand. I know I should not have tried to pick up the carton with my left hand, so I placed my wallet and keys on a refrigerator shelf while shifting the carton to my right hand. One huge problem was I forgot to retrieve them. The following morning, I *was* (key word being, *was*) going out to breakfast with a friend and discovered my wallet and keys were not in the drawer where I always placed them. I spent a couple of hours searching, only to find them by accident when I opened the refrigerator to make a sandwich for lunch. I blamed my stroke, while my brother, Edward, teasingly blamed my age.

Out of an abundance of caution, I completed a formal driver's road test before driving again to ensure I remained qualified and was safe for myself and others. One evening, I pulled into a gas station to fill the gas tank and exited the car without turning off the engine. Fortunately, I put the car in park. Then, I unhooked the nozzle, and for a pico-second thought, *What is wrong with this picture?*

- I had not turned off the engine.
- I did not pay cash first.
- I did not unscrew the gas cap.
- I had not selected the desired octane grade.

So, I put away the nozzle and started over by turning off the engine. Sure, I passed the driver's test, but sequencing the process of filling the car with gas was not part of the test! I took note of this sequencing moment without initial concern.

CHAPTER 11:
THE BENEFITS OF MUSIC

I went to a casino to play Black Jack with friends from mid-morning to late evening, something we have done many times before. I am usually a decent player, but that day I lost all my money in eight minutes because I could not think or sequence fast enough, so I made poor decisions. I refused to go to the ATM and withdraw additional money, choosing to walk the casino grounds inside and out and people-watched in both settings for the next eight and a half hours. When we met for dinner, we went around the table, reporting how we were doing. I only mentioned, "So far, the day's gambling has been awful." No one asked me to explain, so I did not elaborate.

· · ● · ·

I am learning how to play the piano though I am not musically inclined. I know how to appreciate it and love trying to make music now. I'm studying from an accomplished musician and piano instructor, Diana, who is a saint with an endless amount of patience in trying to teach me. Post-stroke, I am slower in processing my lessons and practice, even experiencing occasional random sequencing issues or needing to be taught the same lesson or instruction a few extra times for things to fall into place and learn. Trying to keep my fingers and brain in sync can be frustrating or funny. Diana and I share laughable moments as I try to make music, saying to her, "This awfulness is not stroke-related; I just do not have talent!" I absolutely love learning how to play the piano; learning to play and attempting to make beautiful music has been a lifelong dream. I may lag behind, but I am thankful to be able to pursue this dream. It is also an excellent brain exercise despite my dog howling alongside of me when I practice at home. Now and then, I tickle the ivories into music, allowing Diana to remove her earplugs and listen.

Learning to play an instrument and reading musical notes has proven to be beneficial for improving cognitive functions, mood, and quality of life. *Flint Rehabilitation* had an article entitled, "The Healing Power of Music." Researchers published an article in a journal entitled *Brain*. It showed that listening to music for an hour each day improved memory, attention, and mood during the early stages of stroke recovery. Listening to music stimulated structural changes in the areas of the brain responsible for verbal memory, language skills, and focused attention.

In another article in AARP's Bulletin by Neuroscientist Julene Johnson, she wrote about the role of music in cultivating a healthy brain from research and experiences. Ms. Johnson researches cognitive neuroscience and aging. She stated in one of her answers that she observed an older woman with dementia suddenly start playing the piano at an adult daycare center.

"Everyone in the room came to life, moving and tapping their feet and dancing. I was struck by how impactful a tune had on the whole room." She also pointed out that people don't realize the positivity that music can have on their ADLs. "There is all of this potential for music to help improve lives. We've known for centuries that music has healthy benefits going back to early philosophers and thinkers."

Ms. Johnson realizes there is so much more to learn, noting that the National Institute of Health had a five-year research project to accelerate studies about music and dementia. Ms. Johnson's studies of music history and health have proven music's ability was often preserved in people who had a stroke and could not speak, yet they could sing. That finding sparked research to learn what it is about music that is so special in the context of brain injury and disease—how music is preserved when language is not." According to the American Music Therapy Association, "music therapy interventions can address a variety of healthcare and educational goals."

My friend, Jeff, says, "Music often reminds people of a place and time in their lives. We often associate music with great memories, and it can be healing." I love most all music. It can put me in an assortment of moods and indeed reminds me of time and places in life. Best of all, it helps me clean the house while I jam to some tunes. Many nights as I retire for the evening, I put on some music and *daydream* as I fall asleep. For several months after my stroke, listening to music was bothersome noise because of my hearing sensitivities. But now music usually ignites my thinking and has a calming effect on me. I was *bummed out* for a while until I could appreciate music again.

My physical functions took a huge hit to the point of initially having no leg functionality. Then gradually, I obtained partial recovery through rehabilitation therapies. Later, I was able to perform exercises to learn how to walk again. Today, some physical functions remain slightly challenging. Lifting, gripping, or moving objects might take a little extra concentration and carefulness to complete. Even though I am better able to compensate for these actions, I don't dare handle anything breakable or of sentimental value because if I drop something sentimental, that crashing and breaking sound will mean my sure death! When I hold my baby grandson, I make sure I am seated and pillows surround me.

Holding anything forces me to be more aware and cautious. Though I trust my body more now than ever, I remain very cautious as I still have moments of unsteadiness and spatial issues.

Chapter 12:
Pseudo-Bulbar
Affect (PBA)

G radually, I stopped using a wheelchair, a walker, and my various canes, choosing to walk without assistance as much as possible. I may dust off a cane when going to a busy or crowded place, so people might understand why I walk funny, or at least physically see my deficits. On the rare occasion that I fall, I am a smidgen less embarrassed when someone helps me up, figuring the person sees an apparatus and is less likely to wonder what is wrong with me.

On the day of my discharge from the third hospital, a nurse took Abbey aside and told her to look for changes in me because as we adjusted to my return home, there may be a rough road ahead as we accepted and adjusted to our new circumstances. We had no true gauge of the challenges ahead! Nothing seemed normal after my stroke.

It is very important for me to have order and plans for my day because without some structure, I feel like everything is on the *fly*. I enjoy spontaneous fun time, but I need structure in my day.

I quickly began wondering how other patients seemed so calm and managed their stroke recovery. Neurologists, other doctors, mental health professionals, and especially rehabilitation experts, cautioned me from comparing my stroke recovery to other survivors as each survivor will have different outcomes or results that are unique to his/her stroke event and his/her varying influences, such as the severity of the stroke and any pre-exiting health conditions that factor into a person's overall health before the survivor's stroke event and age, as a few examples.

One survivor may suffer a problem while another survivor is unaffected. Be aware a survivor may have difficulty modifying behaviors to fit varying situations because of a condition known as the Pseudo-Bulbar Affect (PBA). It is a brain condition often causing spontaneous, uncontrolled, emotional reactions whereby the survivor suddenly cries or laughs for no apparent reason. The PBA may cause survivors to have difficulties regulating emotions, finding themselves laughing at a funeral, crying at a joke, showing no emotions at all, or even verbalizing embarrassing or inappropriate comments. Other survivors may not exhibit any symptoms.

According to the American Stroke Association, "After a stroke, survivors often experience a range of emotional and behavioral changes. The reason is simple. Stroke impacts the brain, and the brain controls our behavior and emotions." The changes are a common effect of stroke. "Not only can stroke impact one's mood and outlook, but the area of the brain injury and chemical changes may have significant effects on the brain."

Many symptoms may fall under the PBA, which the American Stroke Organization writes, "When parts of the brain that control emotions are injured, PBA (also called emotional liability or reflex crying) occurs. Most often, people cry easily. Some may laugh uncontrollably or have sudden mood swings. These are physical effects of the stroke. The effects are uncontrollable and can occur without an emotional trigger."

"Another development from stroke or another brain injury may be a lack of empathy, whereby a person appears more self-centered, presenting selfish behavior. This may be because the injury made it more difficult for the survivor to emotionally relate to others. Another side effect of PBA is impulsiveness.

This is characterized as the inability to think ahead or understand consequences. Impulsiveness is more commonly experienced by survivors with right-side or front lobe stroke."

"Individuals with low empathy can sometimes appear aggressive, dismissive, or demanding. If your loved one acts this way to you, don't take it personally. Remember, they are not in complete control. They have a lot more emotions and fewer inhibitions now, compared to before their injury."

"After a stroke, a person may sometimes become less empathetic to others. Empathy means being able to see something from another person's point of view. Without empathy, someone may say or do things that are hurtful to others. A lack of empathy after a stroke is usually upsetting for friends and loved ones but is typically unnoticed by the stroke survivor. It can result in self-centered behavior and damaged relationships."

Very little was the same old me. Before my stroke, I was a reasonable person with a tolerable mix of type A and B personality traits, while balancing home life and a working career I loved like so many others. I understood life's preciousness and joys, doing my best to always remain appreciative in realizing my family's fortunate happiness, health, and well-being. My family will always remain paramount—in particular my desire for a renewed stronger, loving bond with Abbey and my Girlies. Today, I proudly celebrate my Girlies' great successes for what they have built for themselves now and for their futures. They have overcome overwhelming adversities and flourish in life's journey! When they are happy, I am happy!

When my personality completely transformed me into an ugly self after my stroke, dis-inhibition replaced my inherent verbal filtering ability. Dis-inhibition refers to the brain's inability to control or mitigate inappropriate behaviors or impulses and is common for survivors who have sustained a brain injury. My inherent brain filters no longer worked. I had trouble exercising self-restraint over verbal anger, irritability, and impulsive behaviors. I over-reacted first instead of having rational thoughts first, even when I was able to recognize my behaviors were wrong. I was not perfect pre-stroke, but now things were significantly exasperated for the worse. I read numerous medical publications and other online resources that conveyed a repeated theme. Survivors do not believe or mean the hurtful words they may say; this behavior is an impulsive reaction often due to the brain's weakened ability to control inappropriate responses.

A neurologist explained my condition as perhaps two ongoing issues. My negative behavior post-stroke may be the result of neurochemical actions occurring in my brain or a situational stimulus, meaning something in the moment triggers my impulsive, negative reaction.

I responded, "In the interim, family and friends can be tested to their tolerance limits. Granted, everyone should be as patient as possible, but that is a Herculean *ask* of anybody, especially when he/she are being mistreated over a sustained period." Trigger points differ with every survivor, but with enough time, a survivor should naturally regain control.

Today, my impulsive anger has dissipated significantly. Unfortunately, I have momentary flare-ups. Abbey will likely say that my word choice of momentary is subjective, LOL (laugh out loud). I recognize these potential flare-ups faster and try to preempt potential effects and apologize as quickly as possible when I make a mistake. The age-old adage of counting to ten before responding still has merit.

I was NEVER aggressive or violent in behavior! I was verbally angry.

My anxiety level worsened as my behavior remained hurtful. My behavior triggered my anxiety, and the more anxiety-ridden I became, the more my behavior became pronounced and dramatic. The two emotions fed off each other. My anxiety was primarily driven because I had zero understanding of why I had little to no control over emotions, even while recognizing them as flawed. I cried more than my family realized. I was not heartless; I was an ugly new *self.* Compounding issues were my initial refusals to seek outside help other than trying to research post-stroke personality behaviors and hoping to find answers before losing confidence to return to *my true self.* Over all these years, I continually say, "I just cannot believe or understand the brain has that much power over me, over us, ESPECIALLY when capable of recognizing a problem." Self-awareness plays a critical role in our lives at all ages, so I solely blame myself and offer no excuse for my ugly emotional self.

I failed to acknowledge I needed help quickly. Years before my stroke, Abbey and I realized changes in one another but appeared to be mutually committed to ensuring our happiness together. We engaged in many heart-to-heart conversations, which were sincere, productive, and fruitful as we worked through solvable issues, hoping for a lasting resolution. But all bets were off the table once my post-stroke temporary ugly *new self* reared its head.

I respectfully understood Abbey rightfully did not want to be around my anger, let alone continue to work on ourselves. But I was not convinced Abbey truly desired any compromises pre-stroke anyway. I felt dismissed, and my efforts were discounted as I tried to keep us together. Then, as my dis-inhibition lingered, I purposely moved forward, thinking, right or wrong, that my feelings would be heard, and I would no longer be dismissed. It felt liberating, and I stopped working in a concerted effort to make changes with Abbey, but nothing good came from that attitude! Years later, Sara shared with me her meaningful thoughts from her perspective as a young child, wondering, *Did Dad's stroke become the final reason why Mom's and Dad's relationship unfolded? Is Dad grieving his past self and that is why he is so emotionally angry?* Yes, and yes. There is a complicated truth to both of Sara's insights.

When we are in our twenties, no one researches a condition we may suffer from later in life in order to acquire the necessary skill sets to recover efficiently. I had an awareness and cursory knowledge of strokes, taking healthful measures to hopefully ward off ANY potential health problem, but I had no broad understanding of a stroke's many effects. I felt utterly alone in my research to recapture my *normal self* and control my negative behaviors. My well-intended attempts to change were learned daily via trial and error or improvisation. I do not believe you can be taught how to regain your former self, but you can learn how to modify or mitigate varying circumstances. I felt I was in a perpetual survival mode, trying to stay one step ahead of who I became.

A couple of weeks before my overseas war assignments in 2001 and 2002, the medics and my private physician wrote glowing health reports. Then, upon returning from overseas duties, I once again received outstanding follow-up health reports, further proving I was considered to be healthy. I was already completing numerous 5K and 10K charity running events in between my regular exercise routines, completing a

> When I was growing up, my brothers and Uncle Solomon taught me the value of being physically fit and health-conscientious by maintaining an active lifestyle. We participated in many sports activities, including our favorite: boxing. Watching and learning from my brothers and uncle helped me instill a healthy lifestyle at a very young age. I was rarely sick as a child. Fast forward to my working career, I always had terrific medical physicals before going overseas and only occasionally needed a sick day off throughout my wonderful career. I believed my entire lifestyle of regular fitness preempted severe health concerns for the present and future years.

couple of marathons, and a eating a healthy diet of good foods thanks to Abbey. I had no reason to think I was in jeopardy of such a deadly health circumstance.

Much later I had a stroke! All at once, I felt I had aged, not necessarily maturing or becoming wiser, but simply growing older many years ahead of time. I was forty-two, but now I felt so much older and was unable to wrap my head around having a stroke given I was healthy. A neurologist commented, "If not for your great health, you may not have survived the type of stroke you suffered." Ironic? I am healthy, yet I had a stroke? I instantly viewed my stroke as a weakness. Everyone loses the abilities of youth. Usually, this happens a day at a time. Age and the loss of our youthful skills sort of sneak up on each of us. My stroke caused it to be different for me. I aged twenty years in twenty minutes. There was no time to adjust. One day, all things were possible. The next day, I was in a wheelchair.

CHAPTER 13: THE DOMINO EFFECT

Throughout my life, I have always sought affirmation from family and friends as being a good person. That desire took a quantum leap while struggling to be the same *ol' me* after my stroke. I wanted everyone in my life to see I remained the same fully functional and good person. Unfortunately, I was not the same *ol' me*. There is no way to pinpoint any one worse change post-stroke, but being stroke-fatigued nearly daily and having anxieties at heightened levels created a domino effect on how my family's day was going in terms of their happiness and productivity. That's because my emotions were projected unfairly onto them. Another contributing factor depended upon on how significantly my patience level dropped off as the day wore on. Things tended to snowball negatively when I was overtired or overstimulated, so my family wrongly received the brunt of my backlash.

During the summer following my stroke, we traveled to our lake house with my brother, Eldon, and his family. One

> I continue having spontaneous episodes of crying, often unsure what triggers that emotion. Even when I think I have an inkling of the source, I wonder why I cannot filter my reaction. At best, I can mitigate the severity of my crying. My female friends have similar versions of saying, "Having a bawling cry is a healthy and productive outlet."

beautiful afternoon, we were hanging out on the patio when for no known reason, I lost control of my emotions for several minutes. I rushed into the house moments before bursting into BIG childhood tears, forgetting the house windows were open. I bawled for a few minutes and would have continued longer, but my nephew, Scott, came into my room. I was grateful for the welfare check, yet I was humiliated all at once. Scott was fourteen and already a mature young man; now, he was witnessing my weakest moment.

According to Saebo, Inc.,

> About one-third of all stroke survivors will experience emotional difficulties, and many others may demonstrate personality changes or inappropriate behaviors. These personality changes are subtle for some patients and dramatic for others. In some instances, an individual may become easily irritated or even act out violently.

My disposition at home was vastly different than my temperament at work. Andrea Liner, a licensed clinical psychologist, writes, "It's natural for people to take on slightly different personas at work and at home. After all, our work and home environments place different expectations on us and require us to adapt our behavior." She continues writing, "At work, one likely needs to be viewed as professional, and so you are likely to mute the louder parts of your personality in order to come across as grounded and reliable, whereas at home, we don't fear getting fired for acting and expressing ourselves with our natural selves."

"The workplace typically has a professional environment with defined roles, expectations, and norms. People may adopt a more formal and task-oriented demeanor to fulfill their job responsibilities and meet professional standards. This can lead to a different behavior compared to the relaxed and informal atmosphere of home."

At work, I was abiding by the expectations of professionalism; negative behaviors come with swift penalties. Perhaps the loss of potential promotions, awards, and visible/prime assignments—these may translate into a loss of income. A bad performance report may well have prevented a desired assignment or become disqualified from other jobs at other companies. At home, my penalty was losing my family one step at a time. I lost precious time and bonding opportunities with my family. I lost trust, created discord and confusion, and *amped up* mental health stressors in their lives. Those penalties continue festering within me and have been a far worse repercussion of my hurtful behaviors.

"Emotional and behavioral changes are a common effect of stroke. Not only can stroke impact one's mood and outlook, but the area of the brain injury and chemical changes may have significant effects on the brain" (American Stroke Association). It also states,

> You or your loved one may experience feelings of irritability, forgetfulness, carelessness, inattention or confusion. Feelings of fear, frustration, anger, grief, sadness, anxiety and depression are also common. The good news is many disabilities resulting from stroke tend to improve over time. Likewise, behavioral and emotional changes also tend to improve. Time is on your side.

I respectfully offer my perspective as a survivor. I never felt I had the luxury of time as ever being on my side to heal and return to *my normal*. This *new me* was painfully hurting my family and killing me beyond the stroke itself. I was destroying family bonds, causing untold emotional grief, and creating a hostile home. Healing time was my enemy.

I lapsed into this altered person who took over my life. I felt helpless, alone, and misunderstood, very much wanting to throw myself into my family's arms and cry. But I did not want to be seen as weak while trying to maintain a steadfast belief that I am my own best motivator to end this horror and regain my once decent *self.* I did not want to lose my family, yet I kept driving them further away as my verbal anger and irrational behavior frightened them. I was on the brink of plucking their last nerve and arriving at a last chance to make things right: some call it *hitting rock bottom.*

Even though I was fortunate to have the best neurologist, medical teams, rehabilitation, and mental health professionals expertly care for me with devotion and compassion, no one, not even clergy professionals, could have prepared me or my family for the stinging realization of my negative personality change. I learned family could feel a sense of loss or connection with the stroke survivor and grieve similarly to the death of a loved one as they, too, begin to realize and process their loss.

I longed for the day when my Girlies wanted my support again and would love me despite what was happening to us. I needed them to believe in me to recover and put this *hell* behind us. That meant finding a way to regain their love, trust, and comfort. I believed my family forgot or would soon forget the goodness in me without understanding that I was fighting a battle inside me every day. I wanted us to look toward our new dreams and goals, but I was unsure of how to heal myself and family. My self-respect was frail, so it was not going to be an easy accomplishment.

I love my family more than they can possibly imagine! I wanted to continue joyfully providing my Girlies with a head start on life in hopes of setting them up for greater happiness and successes. I also wanted my relationship back with Abbey. She remained beside me during this tragic time, and I will be forever grateful to her. I wanted us to be a happy family again, filled with simple fun, family vacations, and treasured loving memories.

Before my stroke, my Girlies and I enjoyed playing Bronco Rides. My dad invented this rousing strength test for our amusement and fun time when my brothers and I were little boys, and I carried this FUN tradition forward, playing it with my children. I created Fly Fly Go Away, Fling the Kid, and my Girlies created Daddy Dump Truck. WONDERFUL fun! This is the dad I wanted them to remember; those moments and so many more memories and milestones in their lives still make my heart melt.

I proudly cheered and beamed with pride and happiness when my Girlies had sporting events. Abbey's doting enthusiasm and abundance of applause came from her heart and soul. Her eyes sparkled with joy every time she watched them. There is a special bond between Abbey and our daughters that I am proud of yet somewhat jealous of because The LOUD cheers heard from the sidelines at their sporting events were not mine. Oh, I cheered LOUDLY for them from my heart, but a paralyzed vocal cord and weakened second one only produced sound just above a whisper until I was approved for surgery and other procedures such that I could have louder and more understandable speech. I was sad and often frustrated because I could not be heard, saying with great irony, "The silence of my voice resonates louder than my cheering!" Indeed, eventually, I had surgery in hopes of gaining some voice quality. It helped, though not enough, to still be heard clearly and prevent being drowned out by other cheers.

During the summer following my stroke, Jennifer played in a highly competitive field hockey tournament with numerous round-robin games on a sweltering, humid day as a young teenager. Coaches and parents kept the players hydrated and provided cool towels and shade tents. Nonetheless, Jennifer collapsed after playing numerous games, unable to catch her breath, and started hyperventilating. Within moments, several parents ran toward Jennifer, calling out to Abbey to rush over. Abbey ran to Jennifer, whereas I could only walk via my usual serpentine, dizzy fashion using my cane. A huddle of parents had already surrounded Abbey and Jennifer when I arrived. My feeble voice did not lend itself to being heard as I tried to pass through everyone and help Jennifer. I could not even politely move people aside, knowing I could barely balance myself, let alone move others aside. Everyone was barking out instructions as Abbey then carried Jennifer to the team tent to help her while others called an ambulance. I started walking again, trying to reach Jennifer immediately, but could not keep up. My heart sank as I was helpless to assist.

The ambulance crew treated her, and then as an extra precaution, they transported Jennifer to the hospital with Abbey and me driving behind them. Until she slowly began feeling like her *normal* self, we could not relax. Seeing Jennifer need help was scary for her, Abbey, and me. Later that evening, as I replayed the day's event in my mind, it was another fearful reminder of my inability to protect my family given my condition. I could not immediately help Jennifer in her time of need. My fear and anxiety shook me to the core.

· •●· ·

Pre-stroke, my work responsibilities often called for long work hours— twelve, fourteen, and sometimes eighteen hours a day when overseas in support of world events. This meant a higher level of mental stress with added physical wear and tear. So, I was frequently exhausted before adding other responsibilities to my *to-do* list. A huge downfall became sometimes nodding off for a few moments at my Girlies' sports games or tournaments. Abbey shared with me that Jennifer asked her why I attend games if I sometimes doze a few moments during games. That comment shattered my heart. Jennifer had every right to say that to Abbey and be disappointed with me because, while true, I felt the whole picture was not realized. *All they see is me accidentally dozing, not the reasons behind my inadvert action, either pre-or- post-stroke.* During my Girlies' weekend games/tournaments, I NEVER wanted to miss anything, I happily woke up sometimes at 5 AM and completed my pre-stroke marathon training or exercise routine. I finished household needs and whatever had to be done so I could devote the rest of my full-time attention to my Girlies' exciting sports events. EVERY parent faces a balancing act of some sort when there is less of you than there is for the demand.

After my stroke, things were far more difficult. Stroke fatigue is a proven syndrome labeled as Post-Stroke Fatigue Syndrome, (PSF). It is an overwhelming feeling of exhaustion that does not improve with rest. "Many stroke survivors experience overwhelming fatigue, both physically and mentally. Symptoms can include difficulty with self-control, emotions, and memory (The American Stroke Association published). The PSF has been a chief complaint from other survivors I either formally interviewed or engaged others in conversation regarding our commonalities in trying to be whole again.

All three Girlies played travel soccer and add in Jennifer's field hockey, Maura's track, and Sara's softball and most weeknights and weekends after a full work week plus more was tricky keeping pace while still recovering. Most fun weekends took place with all of us packed into our minivan, making longer drives to neighboring counties, even states, which was sometimes taxing for me, but I never wanted to miss a game! I enjoyed watching them play even with pico-second naps and happily doing whatever it took to watch their sporting events.

Ultimately, my explanations did not matter, as any worthy explanation would only sound like an excuse. In hindsight, I should have napped briefly to restore energy, de-stress, and feel revived. I wanted to spend as much time with my family as possible. I LOVED watching them compete.

$$\cdot\,\cdot\,\bullet\,\cdot\,\cdot$$

As part of a hopeful strategy to mitigate bouts of verbal anger, especially as I became tired from the day's events, I asked my family to please stop me when I got angry by hugging me and trying to calm me down. I had hoped by implementing my strategy, their efforts would abruptly call attention to my acting out, and their hugs would quickly diffuse my anger. Maura compared my request to "jumping on a grenade. It took A GREAT DEAL OF EFFORT." I would add courage, a great deal of courage!

Abbey and Maura occasionally tried to stop my ranting by offering a hug, which was unsettling for them. Let's face it, I was an angry person, so it was tremendously unsettling to approach me while being unsure of my reaction. I then turned to my next strategy of walking out of the room to calm myself down however I could. Sometimes, I tried listening to music, watched TV, or simply just sat taking some alone time. It worked to a point. When I returned, most of the time they RIGHTFULLY moved on from the previous moment, creating their fun and happiness. I felt rejoining them would kill their new happy time, so I often retreated rather than regrouping, further isolating myself and being seen as non-caring.

Abbey's and my relationship was crumbling under the stress of my behaviors and our ensuing family challenges. I accepted the lion's share of blame, having failed to recognize my Girlies and Abbey's needs and the impact my stroke had on them. After all, their lives changed as well, undergoing difficult times and traumatic experiences. It was as if I were wearing blinders and seeing the road down a single path. NO EXCUSE! Eventually, Abbey and I reached a state of complete impasse regarding our relationship, rarely having productive discussions; in fact, it was more bickering and defending ourselves than helpful.

I spoke to a mental health professional regarding my failed recognition of my Girlies' needs. She was blunt, offering that parents are often terrible at realizing how a child is adjusting to a situation because parents are too close, maybe even too far, with their emotional involvement. I needed to acknowledge my family's feelings and do more to help them cope, but quite frankly, how could I help them when I could not even help myself? My Girlies were cheated out of critical, impressionable childhood time, and as a family, we were cheated out of loving, wonderful bonding time. Maura shared years later, "When we were growing up, we spent our time taking care of you. I think I was sad that instead of doing Daddy-Daughter runs and other fun activities together, we were cheerleaders for you while you took your first steps out of a wheelchair. It was not the traditional way to create a Daddy-Daughter bond. Now, as an adult, looking back at that time, I realize it was a way to bond, and I am thankful for it."

Jennifer is private by nature, choosing how and when to express her feelings about our crisis then and today, saying, "I set boundaries to protect my mental health." Today, Jennifer is a well-studied professional, a licensed mental health counselor, and an art therapist. She holds other professional credentials. Jennifer's unique, first-hand perspectives on the situation now allow for understanding our crisis from a personal and professional frame of mind.

Maura had trouble thinking and concentrating while in classes at school, becoming genuinely concerned that her grades would slip and that her classmates would witness dramatic changes in her usual upbeat, happy self. Our daughters enjoyed school, their teachers, and solid wonderful friendships. Many of these bonds continue today. They had a good balance of hard work, sports, and extracurricular activities, so it was imperative to maintain some sense of normalcy even though at home they were surrounded by stress. Maura's outlet was writing, whether stories, poems, or thoughts on paper. Writing gave her freedom to express herself.

Sara would internalize her feelings, rarely letting them be known. Sara shared, "My coping mechanisms meant keeping quiet, bottling up emotions, and sleepwalking. I slept-walked all my childhood years due to extreme stress. I was bottled-up, then exploded out like a wind-up-box." Abbey, Jennifer, Maura, and I would sometimes find Sara out of bed wandering around the house; this sleepwalking may indeed be a by-product of internalizing her emotions and stress.

Abbey had so few outlets to be *normal,* having temporarily paused her career and curtailed activities to stay home and assist me. Early on, she frequently tried to reason with me to get help as everyone's quality of life was suffering. I became defensive when questioned about my behavior, letting her know I had no intention of attending any support group or professional mental health therapy. My primary reason was the fear of being around a possible *woe-is-me, pity-party* group and the potential negative scrutiny associated with seeking help. I had a stereotypical impression of depressing sessions versus the more common uplifting, positive people and environment of support groups. I grew up in a generation where counseling was not as accepted as it is today. For my generation, mental health counseling was frowned upon. Today, mental health is better understood with far less stigma associated with it. Solid mental health is a necessity in today's stress and chaos. In my case, an old-fashioned swift kick in the butt to get over it would be what was ordered in past generations.

If my Girlies' were home when I returned from outpatient rehabilitation therapies, their frequent reaction was to race and hide together, maintaining silence, so I might think they were not home. Many nights, Abbey and the Girlies had slumber parties, distancing themselves from me while waiting for me to go to bed.

They frequently went places together in search of fun activities, whether with friends or other family members to relieve stress and have fun away from where I *hung my hat*. Abbey used to take our daughters to the lake house on weekends or simply go out to eat or to the mall. They walked the dog or went to her brother's house saying, "I kept them out of the house so they weren't yelled at or made to feel like they did something wrong. When your behavior got out of control, we would try ignoring you, hoping you would see that your behaviors were inappropriate, but that just poured more fuel on the fire. I cried myself to sleep most nights, just wishing when I woke up, the nightmare would be over. I did my best to ensure the kids remained in all their extra-curricular activities and normal routines, including formal school sports, club sports, school activities, and any healthy outlets to release the frustrations or stress they were going through. The kids felt safe out of the house, and my release was to watch them have fun!"

I recognized none of their actions were mean; they were just trying to be happy. I was isolated and lonely, but I respected why no one wanted to be with me. My heart ached tremendously to be back in their lives.

As the years have gone by, their perspectives have changed, particularly Maura's and Sara's, as they were so much younger. They are now able to look back at our crisis through adult lenses and formulate a mindset with a far greater understanding and an expanded horizon. Collectively, at such young ages, my Girlies coped the best way they could make sense of things and were, forced to grow up quickly. They looked out for one another, often hanging out in a *sister's room*, locking the door, and play-ing music, then dancing and singing. Sister camaraderie—together, they helped each other shape their coping strategies, as well as with the help of school guidance counselors, caring teachers, and many others. They have moved forward positively, stronger, and successfully.

We were forced into an unwanted change after my stroke with Abbey suddenly becoming responsible for all our wants and needs. Before our crises, Abbey and I worked together to raise and enrich our family; afterward, the four of us depended upon her as I struggled to become whole again. I mourned the loss of who I was, wanting affirmation that they remembered the good qualities of my former positive self.

It was evident to Abbey and Jennifer I had changed upon returning home. Maura and Sara understood a narrower view of our new reality. Maura shared with me, "Sara and I have little memories of who you were pre-stroke; we did not know how to differentiate pre-stroke real dad from post-stroke dad." Maura continued, "I was too young to remember who you were before your stroke and to know what consequences to hold you accountable for; I was only in second grade. You form the bonds at that impressionable age. Most kids are bonding with their father during the years of recovery, but I did not have that time. When you recovered well enough, I had to learn how to reconnect with you. I didn't get the chance to do what most fathers and daughters do together."

My misdirected anger was especially harsh on Jennifer, who was about to enter her teenage years, an impressionable, complicated, and awkward transitional period for all pre-teens. They need extra love, feelings of safety, self-assurance, and continued family bonding with supportive parents at all times, let alone during a family crisis. I did not recognize the isolation Jennifer felt until, unfortunately, much later because I was selfishly absorbed and blinded by my recovery needs.

Abbey began describing my new behaviors as that of Dr. Jekyll and Mr. Hyde, and I fully agreed. I should have stopped doing what I knew was hurtful and wrong. It is not a difficult concept to grasp! Yet, it was as though a switch in my brain turned irrational behaviors on or off with no rhyme or reason.

Alex Shulman wrote an article for *Parade Magazine,* in which she wrote about her husband who had suffered a brain injury after a fall. "Often, when he feels frustrated or threatened, he'll curse and shout and sometimes throw things. This dis-inhibition, as doctors call it, is often a symptom of brain disease, whether from injury or Alzheimer's." She also wrote, "When you feel you are under attack, it's hard to [know how to] react. Truly accepting my husband's agitation as beyond his control enables me to remain calm. I've learned from experience that resistance can make things worse while understanding dissipates resentment and makes things better."

On a personal level, I wasn't ready to take initiatives regarding one-on-one counseling, having been soured by a mental health counselor assigned to my case while enrolled in a private stroke rehabilitation facility weeks after being discharged from all initial hospitals. The ultimate deciding factor not to attend counseling occurred when a so-called professional thought I would simply let one of my Girlies attend private counseling sessions at an unknown, unproven facility without Abbey or me completing research and due diligence on the suggested practice regarding their clientele the facility caters to or their staff counselors. When I defended my point of view, I was seen as being insensitive for not immediately agreeing with Abbey and this unprofessional counselor; I began using this term in my references to the person. Worse, I was darned for trying to research and ensure a safe environment for my daughter. I did not trust or feel comfortable with this unprofessional who dismissed and discounted my concern rather than viewing it as a normal process of protecting our daughter. To this very day, I wish I had been stern with the unprofessional counselor and Abbey on how I felt. Instead, I backed off from my viewpoint, fearing Abbey and my daughter would think my intended protection was just another behavior flaw, and I was being insensitive.

I spoke to my primary care doctor about potential medications that might take the edge off my negative behavior and wild mood swings. I was fearful of taking any medications for concerns I might rely on them to always help me, versus working to help myself. I just wanted something to help ease the anger. At first, I experimented with vitamins and herbals with my primary care doctor's knowledge and consent but then quickly moved onto prescribed medications. I was concerned with being on too many medications at the same time because I was tired or lethargic most times and being athletic again was at the forefront of my mind. I wanted vitamins, not medications.

· • ● • ·

While still living at the third hospital, one morning during my speech therapy exercises, I was told my vocal cords probably would never heal. Rather than accept the newest challenge, I dwelled on its negativity, choosing to feel sorry for myself but hopeful that I would rebound later with a better mental attitude. Shortly after the session, my heart began pounding, my mind raced with *what-if* thoughts, my breathing was a tad more labored, and I became immensely fidgety, wanting to get out of my wheelchair and pace around the room to release energy. Luckily, Abbey was coming to visit me soon and could calm me down. I couldn't wait! Just being with her meant everything to me. But, before her arrival, I sunk deep into pessimistic thoughts and disengaged from the day.

A doctor who was familiar with my case happened to cross my room, waved hello, and then came inside, sensing something was wrong. I suspect this was because I usually gave big hellos and smiles when seeing the staff, but this time, I was noticeably quiet. I mentioned I had difficulty controlling racing thoughts, worried thoughts, and felt very tired even though I had a restful night's sleep. I was panicked, fidgety, and did not want to be *in the day*. I rarely complained, so he took time to talk to me even though he was now diverted from his main task. He tried to calm me and then prescribed a very mild sedative to help ease my anxiety, assessing I was experiencing my first anxiety attack. Pre-stroke, I doubt I experienced anything other than *everyday* concerns or worries. I certainly never had a panic attack and probably could not have defined one either. Today, anxiety and its attacks may become crippling if I do not quickly recognize I am having one and can gain control before it *kicks in*. We worked to understand what triggered these symptoms and how to reset my emotions.

Over time, I had medicines for standard treatments after stroke plus medicine for mood swings thought to be depression, medicine to control panic attacks, muscle twitching, restlessness, and medications for *this and that*. As the saying goes, better living through chemistry!

• • ● • •

At times, the drugs were worse than the stroke itself. I was always tired, brain-fogged, and constipated. Differentiating what was stroke-related concerns and what was medicine-induced was challenging. I believe the best medicine is what NO doctor can prescribe—maintaining a positive attitude and having the ability to laugh at yourself, even cry. These can mitigate the rough moments. I eventually asked the doctors to reduce the dose or eliminate the medicines I was taking in hopes of changing my recovery path. I firmly believe in taking medicine as needed, but you also have to help yourself. Your attitude plays a significant role.

I absolutely needed medications, but some gave me a false sense of comfort in my efforts to heal. I also needed to "pull myself up by the bootstraps," as the saying goes, rather than depend upon other people to make my day. I had to keep a positive mindset, be accountable for a healthy recovery, and, priority one, stop hurting my family. Once off several drugs, with doctors' approvals, of course, I worked to re-focus attention back on how truly fortunate I was despite having a stroke. But the ugliness always lurked somewhere *around the corner.* No prescription drugs or therapy will repair the damage I caused my family. Though I have made great strides in regaining my usual *self,* many days remain filled with past reflections and regrets. I continually adjust and tweak my coping strategies to experience all the happiness of my growing family, friends, life's wonders, and now retirement.

One component of my total ugliness remains my acute sensitivity to what I interpret as disturbing noise. These noises now play a significant contributing factor to my ugly anger, and I cringe when hearing them. Most notably are loud chewing of food; someone's fork stabbing their food as if spearfishing; the constant unraveling of snack/chip bags; loud voices inside a vehicle; revving engines, motorcycles; and the banging, clanging or screeching of anything. These may be normal sounds to others, but they often torture me. I would yell at my family if I heard anyone loudly placing her silverware back on the meal plate instead of softly setting it back down. I am hyper-sensitive to what I perceive as noise and recognize this hearing sensitivity is my problem, so I do not expect anyone to understand or take measures to mitigate my problem. I asked my neurologist and even other primary doctors if my poor handling of varying noises is a direct result of my stroke. Sadly, the answers have always been "Yes." I frequently wear earplugs now and, while they may not be fashionable, no one wants to punch me in my face as I cringe because of noise made by him/her.

Over the years, no significant improvement has occurred in my ability to interpret varying sounds as normal to help tolerate the perceived noise. In fact, I may be worse according to Abbey. I continue cringing and dare to complain whether Abbey is assembling household items, fixing things around the house, hanging decorations on the walls, or so kindly cooking delicious meals while banging pots and pans and dishes along the way. I sometimes complain of these *disturbing noises, so* more than once, Abbey has playfully directed a hammer or pot toward me. I am surprised one of them has not found its way to my forehead!

> Car rides with passengers having simultaneous conversations are sometimes challenging because keeping pace and processing varying information is difficult. If someone is speaking fast, I have to ask her/him to repeat what was said. I am on a *seven-second radio delay,* I tell folks, trying to mingle humor in with my request. If anyone is chewing gum or eating crunchy foods, and I hear it. It is double auditory overload trouble, so earplugs are my *go to* solution.

Family dinners should always be pleasant, not just because of the enjoyable meal but also because of the conversations going around the table. We used to mimic a scene from a movie, whereby we went around the dinner table sharing our highs and lows of the day. Fun! But the scraping, clanking, or stabbing of food, general kitchen noises, and fast conversations across the table became overwhelming as my ears interpreted things as painful *noises* rather than the pleasantries of family dinner time. When the noise bothered me, Abbey would say, "We are not doing anything wrong." Indeed, they were not doing anything wrong. My irrational behavior filled the air with tension, a very low point.

One evening at the dinner table, I was on sensory overload from the normal events of the day. I was tired, oddly emotional, and had a headache. Needless to say, I was cranky, irritable, and less than polite in telling them to be mindful of my noise sensitivity. The four of them could no longer hold back their frustration with me, so they put aside their silverware and began eating our comfort meal of hot dogs without the buns, mixed with ketchup, mustard, baked beans in sauce, corn, and peas with their fingers (a sloppy mess!) to avoid being harassed over common noises and to make a *point.*

I had to smile inwardly and applaud them because they humorously made a valid, in-your-face point, while it was so heartbreaking all at once!

Many evenings, I did not join family dinners. My rationale was to give them a happy, peaceful time together without spoiling their evening. I believed I was doing the *right thing*, but it produced a different cause and effect. My action further spiraled me into isolation and feeling awful for losing precious family bonding time.

•‧●‧•

I have difficulty summing up our years of struggles. As I continued working on recovering my real self, I had to find a way to move past my grief, my anger at having a stroke, and my disappointments of not recovering fast enough to help my family and myself. I was not the role model I wanted to be in turning my stroke into a life lesson on how to gracefully cope and work through a life-altering event.

CHAPTER 14:
A LONG, HARD LESSON

The *American Stroke Association* published an article entitled, "Together to End Stroke," where it states, "The loss of a person's former identity and the grieving process are closely linked and can take many forms, including depression, irritability, anger, anxiety, and apathy." Mental health counselors at my hospitals included shock, denial, anger, bargaining, depression, testing, and acceptance. The grieving process is a way for people to heal after experiencing loss.

I believe any identity or personality change can be difficult for stroke survivors, their family members, and even their caregivers to accept. Health care professionals at all my hospitals did not know me pre-stroke and, therefore, could only assess my mental health based on their observations in a controlled hospital environment. It was not until I returned to real-world environments and living that my *new self* rear its ugly head.

I was learning who I was. I was trying to heal quickly, develop strategies to defeat my ugly behaviors, and create a new future in the event I did not fully recover. As my family grew unsure of me and their future, they became less tolerant of my *ANGRY new me,* I never felt so misunderstood or lonely as I did at that point in my life, and it was not anyone's fault.

The grief and guilt of hurting my family handicapped me more so than any lingering limitation or deficit today. The pain I caused and the consequences of our collective experiences are the most challenging day-to-day rehabilitation efforts I continue to face. During our family crises, when I looked in a mirror, I had to remind myself this *new me* is temporary; this is not at all how I behave or who I am. I will always be ashamed for projecting my anger onto my family. Sadly, I had no coping skills or mechanisms in place to face this challenge, relying heavily upon being able to own my recovery under my terms to return to being a nice guy. Caring people in my world would say things that were warmhearted: "Go easy on yourself. Take things one day at a time. The best is yet to come." All well-intended comments, but I needed tangible, actionable skills.

My father and aunt had strokes, initially managing their recovery health and emotions. Eventually, both required constant care and helpful cues to communicate. Sadly, at some points, it seemed they were a prisoner in their own bodies, reduced to far less than their usual, vibrant, working selves. Witnessing their deterioration is a reminder of what could have happened to me, while suffering the same fate. I often look back at their struggles and wish I knew then what I know now to better understand what they were going through to have helped them more.

I viewed myself as a recovery failure in the first fifteen months back home and believed my family would agree, so I voluntarily left the house without first discussing anything with Abbey or my Girlies. I simply gathered my clothes and a few belongings and departed, figuring no one would truly care. I thought some time away from the family would allow them to heal, have normalcy in their lives, and give me a renewed perspective on recovering. Hopefully, the time away would allow us to refresh our realities, then lead to eventual reconciliations. I moved out of town into my brother Edward's home, hoping to use the time away to *fix* myself and be surrounded by a less hurried atmosphere. I continued my visual meditation, visualizing myself with my family, my Girlies' at their events, whether sports, school, or any event they were involved in, I envisioned having fun during a weekend or simply picnics. I envisioned what life looked like after I healed. I joked with Edward, saying we should build a Star Trek Holodeck to create the scene and let me live these visions in the Holodeck until I healed and the moments could become real again.

Abbey and I were separated for just over two years, and I avoided many of our mutual friends during that time. I fully credit Abbey with ensuring we had opportunities for family events together, regardless of which side of the family was hosting an event. She periodically invited me over for dinner to hopefully enjoy family dinners again. But she was not interested in trying to go out on a date, so a second courtship appeared out of the question until I sought outside help and could prove my *goodness* was permanent. I stubbornly continued refusing help, defending myself to regain discipline and restrain angry outbursts. Mental health counseling was easily accessible during my hospital stays, but at that exact moment in time, I did not know about this terrible *new me* nor did any medical personnel. I was an easygoing patient, not needing or wanting anything but the continued kindness and expertise of staff to help me while I was solely focused on rehabilitation healing. I never knew a change in personality was possible after a stroke.

During our long separation, I had many distractions in the mornings and afternoons between work, personal routines, and *doing life.* I was busy and distracted during the day, but nighttime was lonely, having fewer distractions. I usually stayed awake, distracting myself by reading, watching television, or listening to music until I could no longer hold my eyes open to avoid lying in bed replaying our family struggles that I caused. I promised myself tomorrow would be better than relaxed— hoping to fall asleep quickly.

Abbey and Jennifer were skeptical about me rejoining the family when I thought I was ready to return home full-time without obtaining help first. I ached so very much to be in their lives full-time again and not just when we would visit each other. Abbey, Maura, and Sara made every effort to maintain some sense of normalcy during our two-year separation. Maura and Sara visited me many weekends, whether for the day or overnight, and I ensured they were comfortable and had fun. However, Jennifer was justifiably distant, keeping her guard up. Her absence tore me up. I was losing her, if not already having lost her. I tried to understand her need to socialize with friends and do things she wished for as a budding teenager, but more often than not, I felt pushed away.

Jennifer was now officially a teenager, so her distancing could have been the normal growth and mindset of wanting to spread her wings, have a social life of her choosing, and gain even more independence. Teenagers do not necessarily want to hang out with their parents as they struggle to find their place in the world. So, how much of Jennifer's distance was a reaction toward my ugliness, and how much was being a typical teenager? Right or wrong, my mind said her absence resulted from her not wanting to be with me. I was emotionally hurting them and bringing down their positive energy. I could not blame Jennifer if she were mad and no longer trusted me. I respected that. It painfully hurt, but I got it. I caused the family crisis, which complicated everyone's world.

Even though I initially left the house voluntarily, collectively, I was not welcomed back now. They were happy being themselves again without *penalty* and feared my return would amount to the same old problems. It was an abrupt reminder that my behavior was the direct opposite of my inspirational intent of showing when life doles out hiccups, you can find a way to endure and overcome. Like Uncle Solomon, finding something good from something so terrible can help *things* normalize with time.

Dr. Gary Seale, Regional Director of Clinical Services for the Centre of Neuro Skills at the Houston and Austin, Texas, clinics wrote, "If you can find the good after stroke, that is resilience!"

I tried to find ways for our family to socialize and bond comfortably. Edward had a great idea to bond with Maura, which sparked loving, memorable times. Maura loves science, particularly planetology. She enjoyed taking her telescope outside to view the sky as a young girl, so Edward suggested we take Maura to the Friday evenings public science lectures at the state university where she would have opportunities to attend these science lectures and then go into the observatory to use their high-powered telescopes. Afterward, we returned to the main building and enjoyed hot chocolate, our favorite treat on chilly nights. We attended these public lectures produced by graduate students reasonably often. One evening a student commented: "How wonderful it is to see Maura attend, taking notes with genuine interest." When the student asked her age, I answered, "Ten." The expression on his face was priceless.

Maura slept over with me at Edward's flat, which I jokingly called his home, one special chilly night. The three of us woke up at 2 AM to view Saturn's Rings at the peak of their seasonal brightness through Maura's telescope and then through Edward's more advanced telescope, while sipping hot chocolate. It was a fun and memorable early morning, and a pleasant start to the day ahead!!

Several friends thought our family crisis experience would strengthen us by bonding and helping each other through our time of need. That would have been possible, but as my anger and frustrations became increasingly unacceptable, I was no longer trusted and now considered a negative *influencer* (a term used today) for so long. My Girlies lost a piece of their childhood innocence just trying to be normal kids, and without a *normal* father, they rightfully relied on Abbey for nearly everything that both parents should have a role in. I felt cast away. Real or imaginary I was in a perpetual spiral of feeling my value to the family diminished. It was how I felt, and feelings are not right or wrong. They are simply about how you feel. Maura sums things up elegantly, "We lost a safe, healthy, home environment."

Years before my stroke, Abbey and I realized changes in one another but appeared to be mutually committed to ensuring our happiness together. We engaged in many heart-to-heart conversations, which were sincere, productive, and fruitful as we worked through solvable issues, hoping for a lasting resolution. But over time, I was no longer convinced Abbey truly desired any compromises as I tried to keep us together despite feeling dismissed, and my efforts to help us were discounted. I appealed to Abbey to recognize efforts and compromises must be a two-way investment. Already on shaky ground, all bets were off the table post-stroke once my temporary ugly *new self* reared its head. I respected that Abbey rightfully did not want to be around my anger, let alone continue to work on ourselves. Then, as my dis-inhibition lingered, I purposely moved forward, thinking right or wrong that my feelings would be heard, and I would no longer be dismissed. It felt liberating, and I stopped working in a concerted effort to make changes with Abbey, but nothing good came from that attitude!

While living with Edward helped, my heart ached so much, wanting to be with my Girlies full time. I began renewed conversations appealing to Abbey to recognize our efforts must be a two-way investment. Abbey wanted more healing time and assurance that changes were made before I returned home. My return depended upon my fulfilling her legitimate conditions, and I wanted her to realize her promised compromises. I readily agreed to many of her requests, but with other unresolved issues lingering, we hit another impasse, so I began preparations for a potential divorce as we grew further apart.

In last-ditch efforts, my Girlies created daughter interventions for Abbey and me, presenting ideas and constructive action plans with poise to help us *right the ship.* They politely but firmly conveyed that we move on as a family unit or divorce. Either way, we must decide soon because our family could not continue living like this. They presented their advice with wisdom well beyond their years, and we were very impressed! Abbey and I were then left alone to reconcile. Unfortunately, we could not come to terms, but we finally agreed to marriage counseling before forging ahead with a divorce. Marriage counseling helped, but our efforts were not sustained as one of us would *suddenly give up* for no apparent reason.

Sara told me years later, now with adult eyes looking back at our time, "You and Mom did not invite us into decision-making conversations, so we did not feel included when decisions were made. We tried interventions and advising you, but nothing proved beneficial, so we decided to *stay out of the middle.* Ultimately, the decisions were made by you two, so why bring things up again?"

Sara also shared her meaningful thoughts from her perspective as a young child, wondering if, "Dad's stroke became the final reason why Mom's and Dad's relationship unfolded? Is Dad grieving his past self, and that is why he is so emotional and angry?" Yes, yes, and yes. There is a complicated truth to all of Sara's insights.

Jennifer, Maura, and Sara prepared a unique, loving picnic intervention for Abbey and me in the side yard of our home one pleasant evening. They dressed up, acted as our servers, and showed us a means to reconnect and how to be a loving family. That moment is etched in my fond memory bank forever. It was so brilliant of them—so perfectly thoughtful! Abbey's reason for not filing for a divorce remains her love. She said, "Having grown apart by different ideals, goals, and visions of a future together as we have aged, our unexplainable *link* keeps us together; it may be because we *have* each other's backs, and that is unbreakable to me. We have both given up a great deal for one another and have a shared history and beautiful memories together."

•• ● ••

We tried healing our family unit via as many productive means as possible despite it all. Abbey learned the state charter for the Brain Injury Association of America was holding their annual conference in our city, which she believed may be helpful for us to attend. Their charter mission states, "They are the voice of those affected by brain injury through advocacy, education, and research." Their vision is to, "Bring health, hope, and healing to those living with brain injury, their families, and the professionals who serve them."

We attended their impressive multi-day conference, learning a great deal through their resources, listening to keynote speakers, and meeting people experiencing the same concerns as we were. Abbey and I chose to attend a mother-daughter venue regarding how their husband/father drastically changed after his stroke. Before his stroke, they described him as a kind, loving, gentle, man. It was clear they loved him with great passion, but he became an overbearing, mean bastard post-stroke.

The wife and daughter stood by him for as long as possible, eventually leaving because they could no longer tolerate his acting out in such a negative manner. Their stories of dealing with him were so heartbreaking. I cried during their presentation, feeling sorry for them, as well as seeing myself and what I was doing to my family. I looked at Abbey at the end of their speech and cried even more, knowing no apology could do justice to how I wanted to make peace at home.

In my conversations with other stroke survivors whether through my interviews, attending survivor events, or my stroke support group, they have shared stories of their feelings and uncertainties soon after their strokes. One person described his stroke as an opportunity to learn new things and allow himself to inspire new thoughts of creativity. Another was thankful he was left in-tact, still with abilities to perform most everything as before his stroke. Another survivor was fascinated at the process of learning to walk again stating, "How did we learn as babies? I have all these pulleys, straps, and apparatus now to help me stabilize and balance." Others were thankful and focused on capabilities that remained, not what was taken away from them.

While many days remain an emotional roller coaster ride, I am keenly aware I should not complain, given the unfortunate reminders of how much worse I could be as seen in other people's recovery trials and tribulations—as soldiers, innocent children, or any number of survivors.

Chapter 15:
The Value of a
Strong Family

Doctor Nicole Andretta, Director of Rehabilitation Centre for Neuro Skills in San Francisco, wrote of patients learning what strengths and wisdom they have drawn from their stroke experience and trying to help them build behavioral tools and finding hope. She also spoke of families or friends fracturing or coming together after a stroke, commenting that brain injury recovery is hard work requiring skilled therapists to help. She emphasized that the brain and human spirit are amazing in their ability to heal.

Looking at past years via wonderful family photographs or videos can be extremely emotional because it reminds me of time gone by, seemingly so fast, and also of what I had or damaged. The photos are of happy times I wish hadn't been paused because of my stroke. Looking at photos should always be joyful, but for me, post stroke, it is a reminder of no longer getting that time back again.

Luke Russert, son of national newsman/reporter Tim Russert, quoted his father as saying, "When my life is over, there's nothing more I'll be judged on than what kind of father I was." Mr. Tim Russert conveyed a powerful sentiment I also believe. Regardless of the kindness I spread while working around the world during my former career or the proud accomplishments I achieved via other means, during the most difficult time in our lives, I wanted my Girlies to judge me on the totality of the person I am, not just me as a father. ALSO, I wanted to show my family that we could face adversity head-on and still find something good. I wanted my Girlies to remember that about their great Uncle Solomon and wanted them to see that characteristic in me as well. Abbey and I taught them about their elders of pastgenerations, so they knew where they came from and who they are now because of other family mentors before them. So many elders passed to their eternal bliss before my Girlies had a chance to meet them. In some cases, they passed away just a few months before or after they were born.If they had time, or more time together, it would have had a substantial positive impact on my Girlies.

I made numerous mistakes during my recovery journey, bringing pain into my Girlies' lives and my marriage. I lost sight of using this event as a positive *teaching moment:* When life hiccups on your plans, you will find inner strength to heal all.

I carry the weight of immense guilt for having been such an SOB during our excruciating *dark* period. I have moved past the stroke, itself, *but* the shameful ugliness of my behaviors will always be my enduring deficit/ pain. Today and always, it is a critical balancing act for me to remain focused on the positive, mitigating the negative, and concentrating on how thankful I am to be with Abbey, Jennifer, Maura, and Sara. Each day is an extra day to hug and kiss them, let them know they are loved, and show how proud I am of them. I recognize more than ever the value of a strong family.

Chapter 16:
My Recovery

A former support group facilitator began using the term *improve, improving,* or *improvement* rather than the word *recovery* to describe our journey. As casually mentioned to me, "This is slowly becoming a way of thought—you improve after your stroke or brain injury, but the effects remain during your lifetime. The thought behind this movement/change appears to be the now belief that stroke effects will always remain, so the survivor will improve but not fully recover.

Abbey and my Girlies played critical roles in my recovery. Their combined engagement sparked my exercise regimen and connected us at a time when we were desperate for positive moments. I did not always thank my family for their special ways of caring for me; however, I am very cognizant that my achievements are because of their steadfast participation in my recovery! It warmed my heart to reconnect with my family, even if only for a few hours. Abbey would comment on how well I was doing or lift my spirits on those rough days of my therapy sessions. She was genuinely there for me whenever I needed her. Abbey had the unpleasant caretaking responsibility of having to wipe my *tush,* and many other experiences we wish to forget when I couldn't easily squat, stand, walk, or have moments of muscle spasticity. Talk about genuinely being there for me whenever I needed her!

Fortunately, I had been remarkably healthy all my life, so I was not used to burdening others. The guilt of relying on others was difficult for me to accept initially, but I required at least some help until I regained abilities, regained confidence, and figured out how to do something in a different manner than the way I did it before my stroke. My self-esteem was very fragile immediately after my stroke, and, quite frankly, it remains somewhat fragile as I am reminded that I cannot do things as before.

A very powerful quote of the day came from an online posting of *Flint Rehab's*: "Progress might not always be easy or visible, but with the right tools and mindset, it's absolutely possible."

My recovery is an on-going process as I am fortunate to continue slowly improving even nearly twenty years beyond my initial stroke event. I am thankful for a continued team of medical professionals and rehabilitation therapists, past and present, who still advise me during all phases of my journey. I am convinced survivors need active family support, solid friends, and other supportive people to help her/him achieve maximum recovery goals. I need to feel a part of the medical management team because, I believe, the medical team can only take a survivor so far without the survivor's genuine participation. It is a mutual effort toward moving forward and optimizing recovery goals.

I learned from personal experience that recovery is not strictly repairing physical damage; there was also emotional damage to heal for me AND my family. Family, and the numerous stories I have heard while attending stroke support groups, remind me that your loved ones, even caregivers, experience emotional stages while caring for someone. Immediately after my stroke, I had to have faith in my abilities to improve and ensure I looked positively toward tomorrow, asking myself, *What can I do today to make tomorrow easier?* I knew if I did not stay positive, the path toward a meaningful recovery would be lost. My very first steps in physically recovering were to first learn patience, then maintain a never-give-up-hope attitude, no matter how long my journey. Time and its results were very scary unknowns. I had to put in maximum positive efforts and then have the strength to accept the outcome, even if it were a potential negative result. This was easier said in my head than actually doing it. Consistently staying positive, believing in myself, and giving some things up to fate AND faith were sometimes harder than doing my rehabilitation exercises.

I also learned it was *one thing* to learn a skill at the hospital, but *another thing* to come home, requiring assistance for nearly everything, including needing Abbey to clean my tush after using the bathroom. We all need help, and I respect that. It just was not easy to *wrap my head around* that I needed the help.

Days after my stroke, I asked a few specialists caring for me why did I have a stroke, often mentioning my active lifestyle and fortunate good health all my life. I enjoyed fitness workouts, a variety of sporting activities, and a healthy regimen. One doctor said the best thing I could to do for myself was to stop questioning the reason I had a stroke despite my fitness regimen and *move on,* maybe never knowing why. Some might say that was tough love; for me, his comment was the beginning of trying to understand my fate and concentrate on day-to-day healing targets. Long-term goals outside my stroke care were paused if not directly related to my immediate healing quest. It was a bit unsettling not knowing if any function would return, and if some did return, how long would it be before I regained them. Patience is not my best quality. I wanted to be healthy now! Moving on allowed me to accept that recovery did not have to be sweeping all at once. I could go forward with a sincere effort to improve and believe in myself. I had to work hard and then have confidence to let God decide my fate beyond what I could do for myself. Whatever progress I could achieve (maybe none), I had to find happiness and recognize my courageous efforts. As the saying goes, "An inch is a cinch, a yard is hard." I worked to the best of my ability!

At first, fear motivated my desire to heal quickly rather than determination. Fears of not returning to my *normal* and fears of whatever deficits remain will only get worse in my later years were not productive. Each survivor should determine what methods work for him/her to increase the possibility of recovering from stroke paralysis. It might not be easy, so please note whatever your motivating factor, it helps to be surrounded by supporting family and friends. I worked and tweaked efforts to find a means to remain continually motivated in pursuit of my healing goals. There is no fairy dust to sprinkle; I knew I was going to have to work to achieve maximum results and capabilities in restoring my health. I handled aspects of my healing journey terribly, fraught with pitfalls, learning moments, and an abundance of mistakes. However, I did whatever I could to regain my body when it came to exercise and therapies. I pushed myself, spoke in depth to other survivors, had enlightening conversations with clergy and religious friends, persevered through a never-give-up attitude, and trusted God more than ever. Every survivor's journey is different; no two shall be the same. My friend, JW," summed up his stroke journey by saying, "I am not who I was anymore, but who I am still matters." That is a powerful reflection! JW's and my journey may differ, but our mindsets and thoughts are the same.

Many decades ago, scientists believed the brain had a limited number of brain cells that faded or died off as we grew older. This has proven to be untrue; the brain is indeed fluid and is able to rewire itself throughout our lives via neuroplasticity, the brain's ability to form and reorganize synaptic connections, especially in response to learning something new or from your life experiences. Through repetition of an action, exercise or via your experiences, the brain's pathway is reinforced, strengthened or is able to form new pathways and connections to deliver messages.

Synaptic connections are the connections between neurons that allow them to communicate with each other and transmit information to the brain for processing (*Flint Rehab*). "The human brain can change and heal at any age, any time, not just in its recovery stage, thanks to neuroplasticity. This incredible process allows our brain to continuously adapt, heal, and create new pathways that are crucial for cognitive and motor skills." Neuroplasticity is explained in the following way: "When a street or freeway entrance has been blocked along your daily commute, the GPS may suggest an alternative route. This alternative route may be unfamiliar and take longer to navigate, but it will still lead you to your destination."

Medical professionals know so much more now than two decades ago, even since 2015. These advances, including new data, are taking the field in a new direction and of stroke management. Again, my stroke was in 2005, still at the point of great research and data being compiled particularly from soldiers returning from the Iraq and Afghanistan wars. Today, there is so much published information in a variety of sources regarding stroke and its subtopics. A stroke support group buddy, Jeff, looks at his recovery efforts this way: "I may be different, but only because it is harder for me to do things the way I did so before my stroke. I get the job done, just differently." It may take Jeff extra time, but he does not give up, knowing he will continue to improve.

While many stroke survivors might not achieve a full recovery, functional gains are possible with the right approach and circumstances, experiencing the fastest results during the first few months of recovery when their brain is in a heightened state of plasticity (meaning your brain is trying really hard to recover). After the first three months, progress starts to slow down. This is considered a plateau, and it is not a sign that you should give up. It's a sign that you need to double down. Recovery won't stop as long as you don't stop. Experiencing a plateau or an occasional regression is to be expected. You can move past these setbacks by staying consistent with your rehabilitation program. At the beginning of my rehabilitation process, reaching these plateaus was initially scary because I did not know if I had hit a permanent wall or simply a minor pause. Fortunately, being so athletic much of my pre-stroke life allowed me to understand that these pauses were, indeed, just a pause and the rest the body needed. My plateaus only lasted a week or two, but in the interim, it was nerve-racking not knowing if I had achieved my full potential or the best I would be from here on out (*Flint Rehab*).

"If I survive into my 70s, will it be difficult for my healthcare providers to distinguish between problems caused by my old stroke and normal aging issues?" I think about Carol Keegan's statement often because when I experience minor forgetfulness today, I wonder how much may indeed be a by-product of my growing older, perhaps distractions, or could it be stroke-related?

• • ● • •

Exercises and therapies played a vital role in helping me regain my normal. However, I do not want to downplay the criticality of a strong positive attitude playing a role in recovery. As I gained more strength and better movement in my limbs, I cautiously *raised the bar* of my hopes and expectations, trying to push the limits. Any gain, small or large, fed my motivation, which led to greater self-esteem, optimism for the future, and a sense of accomplishment. I firmly believe doing my Activities of Daily Living is constant therapy, teaching my brain and body how to connect in working together. I try to do all things unassisted, within reason, whether that is going downstairs, reaching for something, and walking easier trails and more because I feel the only way to get better is to try. Maybe I succeed; maybe I don't, but at least I try.

All recoveries come with its ups and downs, so it is critical to stay mentally strong as well. Eventually, I followed up with my mental health well-being despite how uncomfortable expressing myself was beyond time already spent with stroke professionals, while infirmed at the hospital rehabilitation facilities.

Weightlifting/training remains one of my favorite sporting exercises, but I do not have an equal amount of strength in my left arm or leg as compared to my right-side post-stroke. My left side remains noticeably weaker, so certain activities, even holding any object in my left hand, can be tricky. Weightlifting helps restore muscle activity, gain strength, force coordination of body movements, and use proper balance techniques to complete the motion of the repetition. Today, I incorporate weight training as one of my rehabilitation tools for both mental and physical well-being. I like to *hit* the gym in the early morning because it invigorates the start of my day, and usually, there are fewer people working out in the early part of the day, so I am less embarrassed when my body coordination goes awry.

One morning, I was alone in the gym when a guy walked in and settled down on the free-weight chest bench press, asking me for a *spot.* I felt I could not say no, but I also worried if something were to happen, I may not be able to assist properly. His safety had to be a priority, so I began praying someone, anyone, would walk in and take over. As prayer would have it, another gentleman walked in and took over. Keep in mind that weight training focuses on making muscles stronger, whereas rehabilitation exercises are concentrated on rewiring your brain through greater repetition and muscle memory.

Before doing heavier weights for bicep curls, I was ensuring I could handle the range of motion necessary to conduct a proper repetition with light weights. I placed five pounds on the bar as a test when a couple walked in and heard me cursing because my arms were not yet in sync, trying to stabilize the bar. When I finally got a rhythm going and trusted myself, I acted proud, clearing the five pounds on the bar with bravado and having a big smile on my face! I can only imagine what they were thinking.

According to *Flint Rehab* and a variety of other resources I've read, "Chess, Sudoku, crossword puzzles and other brain stimulating games are great for activating the left side of the brain and improving problem-solving skills. Crossword puzzles are especially helpful for developing word recall skills." I've read that board games and card games help us think deeper and help us to regain memory.

> Video games can serve as an effective form of rehabilitative therapy for stroke survivors. To promote recovery after stroke, individuals must play games that engage the skills that were affected by their stroke. For example, if a stroke affects memory, individuals must consistently practice video games that engage memory skills. This helps the brain understand that there is a demand for memory functions, and encourages adaptive reorganization of neural circuitry. "Many stroke survivors struggle to stay motivated and perform the repetitions necessary to influence neurological adaptations. Using video games for stroke patients can help individuals stay engaged and challenged enough to keep practicing. (*Flint Rehab*)

· • ● • ·

My father taught my brothers and me the excellent strategic game of chess at age five: simply learning the names of the pieces first: then later learning how they move; and still later, simple offensive and defensive moves and strategies. Over fifty-seven years later, I still love playing chess with my brother

Eldon, as a chess club member, as an occasional tournament entrant, or with friends, and against the computer. Some of my best memories as a child were crying after I always lost to Dad but then crying happy tears when I rarely beat him or my brothers later in life. Chess combines your ability to formulate strategies and think multiple moves ahead with the reasoning of *if this, then that* consequences. I play chess and other helpful brain games on the computer or the old-fashioned word search print puzzles to exercise my brain. Reading is beneficial as well.

Practicing any form of cognitive exercise helps challenge your brain and assists in forming new neural pathways. It also improves brain health and skills, like memory. *Flint Rehab* suggests the following great exercises by accompanying your caretaker to the grocery store. Allow him/her to tell you to find two or three food items—don't write them down. Once you're able to find these, increase the number to memorize and find. Another exercise is to have your caregiver provide you with two-digit numbers. Add three to this number three times. Subtract seven and repeat. You can also stack coins, use therapy putty exercises, and stretch rubber bands.

My neighbor, Paul, would pick me up to go grocery shopping, which was therapeutic because it gave me buddy time and some laughter as Paul walked me through the aisles using the gait belt. I looked like a dog on a leash, but the looks on people's faces were priceless! Sometimes, I accidentally pushed the cart ahead of us faster than I could walk, then would have to re-balance and bring the cart back inward. It was almost a comedic sight and a gag like we used to watch on old comedy variety shows. One such vignette was Carol Burnett's variety show. I truly did not care what people thought, nor did I care if I made a spectacle of myself. It was both mental and physical therapy for me. I was out of the house, away from the four walls as I called it, my family could relax and breathe easy for a few hours away from me, I was having *buddy time,* and Paul and I could laugh at ourselves, though Paul laughed at me mostly! But laughing at me or with me—it was therapy!

Jennifer filmed moments of my therapies and cheered me on. She also encouraged my desire to participate in stroke survivor charity walks/runs. For a particular charity walk/run, unbeknownst to me, Jennifer created a team made up of family and her wonderful friends to support me and all stroke survivors. She made signs and personalized team T-shirts for us to hold and wear. Go Team Marks! Years later, Jennifer and I went skydiving with family. While she was calm, cool, collected, and looking forward to some air acrobatics, I was NERVOUS, borderline scared! Despite how I felt, I told Jennifer inside the plane I loved this bonding moment and would forever treasure it. Going to the edge of the plane door to get ready for the jump was scary—that is until I reminded myself nothing was scarier for me than my stroke. Suddenly, an eleven-thousand-foot jump seemed like a true adventure!

Part of my regular hospital physical therapy program included kicking or catching a ball and many other hand/eye coordination and balancing exercises. I still could not stand on my own, so a therapist would hold me from behind under my arms as I tried to kick. You gotta laugh; my timing and coordination were way off. I usually playfully blamed the therapist holding me for any errant kicks! I continued these physical rehabilitation exercises upon returning home by asking my Girlies to softly throw me, for example, a tennis ball or foam football to hopefully catch. Unfortunately, sometimes, they heard the sound of my hands clapping, then the sight of the ball smashing my face

Maura enjoyed a fun speech therapy exercise of blowing a cotton ball across a table at one another. Another fun exercise for eye/body coordination was indoor kickball. Granted, we should have played outdoors, but the weather did not always cooperate. We assembled jigsaw puzzles, I taught her some things about the game of chess, and we played *Monopoly* and other board games.

Sara and I played softball in our backyard. We started pitching and catching warm-ups, followed by batting. Well, I was off target most of the time with pitching and batting, giving Sara inadvertent extra exercise by chasing the tennis ball outside of our backyard fence line when I played pitcher. I smiled proudly like a kid in a candy store whenever I pitched inside the strike zone, and we belly-laughed numerous times at my errant pitches. Batting, well, let's just say I needed a great deal of work. Sara, on the other hand, did terrifically. Sara loved softball, and I needed therapy, so we often chose this sport as our fun bonding time.

On a gorgeous fall weekend, we all decided to go outdoors and enjoy some fresh air and fun. I was racing the kids around the cul-de-sac in my wheelchair, just laughing and playing. Unbeknownst to me, Jennifer went inside and brought out the old-fashioned Camcorder of the late 1990s and began filming. In between moments, Jennifer and Abbey completed some fun field hockey practice drills. Maura and Sara were climbing trees and riding bikes when I decided to put on a bike helmet and my gait belt and try walking. Wearing the bike helmet and belt was for dramatic effect, but if I were to fall, there was some semblance of peace of mind to mitigate the possibility of injury. Walking one short baby step at a time gave me the confidence to walk more and show improvement to my family. Jennifer filmed and cheered, Maura and Sara cheered, and Abbey was beside me to ensure I did not go ten toes up. I weebled and wobbled but managed a few yards before she had to grab the gait belt to keep me from falling. It was not pretty to watch, but it did not have to be. I was ecstatic simply trying. My family spent time actively participating in my therapies. No matter what we did together, I was always happiest when I was together with my Girlies. That was my greatest therapy! My heart melts when I am with my Girlies.

CHAPTER 17:
LIFE'S DELICATE BALANCE

The medical and rehabilitation professionals I worked closely with often shared that the brain's ability to adjust is remarkable, emphasizing how effective exercise combined with varying therapies has on the brain. Desiring physical exercise is easy since I have been extremely active all my life. Other key ingredients for my successful recovery were humor and the ability to laugh at myself. I am convinced these, too, helped save my life beyond the support of family, friends, strangers, medical and rehabilitation experts, and God.

Uncle Solomon understood life's delicate balance between good and difficult times. I will always admire his uplifting perspectives and ability to go with life's flow, maintaining his easy-going character and sense of humor. When life became rough, Uncle Solomon remained calm and would somehow find a lighthearted side during a challenging time. You could feed off his strength to calm your own fears. Many times, I was calmed by simply hearing his deep sigh. Then he'd say in a resounding, overly-accented baritone voice, "Evvvvvvveeeerrrythang is gonna be alllllllll riiightttt...but not today." I continually strive to adopt Uncle Solomon's demeanor and strong positive outlook.

Numerous sources agree that exercise improves your quality of life both mentally and physically. However, some survivors may be unable to exercise due to limited abilities. I believe trying is key; work closely with therapists to try and activate muscles. Learn about passive exercises that may stimulate muscles, improve your overall health, and offer hope toward recovering to the fullest potential. Passive exercises are performed with someone, perhaps a machine, manipulating your body for you; someone or something else is conducting the movement. For example, someone raises your arm above your head, then lowers it, and repeats this exercise several times. Passive exercise may stimulate blood flow, provide better circulation, and assist in the process of delivering nutrients and oxygen to body tissue and organs. Even though you are not doing the movement, the passive movement may bring about neuroplasticity. Talk to a doctor or therapist about what is best for you.

If you have some abilities but must take precautions, ask a doctor or therapist for exercises that are best suited for you. Active exercises are physical muscular movements you exert to accomplish something. I had severe trouble with balance, so my therapist provided opportunities to conduct active leg workouts while holding onto my walker, cane, or chair. I did seated marching, leg stretches, toe raises, and an assortment of leg movements while holding onto apparatuses and using therapeutic bands of different degrees of difficulty. I was exercising even while holding onto an apparatus. I was very fortunate to have my strong will and desire to recover and staying faithful to my belief in doing everything I could do for myself first. Then and only then could I ask God for help. I had to help myself first. I needed myself, family, friends, and God to see me sincerely trying everything possible before asking for help to improve. Another key motivation factor was I was only forty-two with so much still possible and a great desire to equally help support and participate with my young Girlies. As mentioned, early in my recovery, I wanted to be seen as a role model; these strong motivation factors helped nurture my diligence to actively participate in rehabilitation. My therapists and I often bonded because they saw I was sincerely working at recovery, thereby providing encouragement and actively participating with me versus just providing instruction on how to complete an exercise. It became a team effort, which further fueled my motivation to try leveling up.

Reaching over my head to get something out of a kitchen cabinet shelf forced me to balance on my tiptoes, hopefully without falling. I had a solid three-second opportunity to do what was necessary, while standing on my tiptoes. After that, failure rates went significantly higher. There was no way to even think of using a step stool, so I turned the kitchen spatula into a handy tool numerous times. I cleaned up a few messes, but then I calculated how close I came to accomplishing my mission before I knocked something over, broke something, or worse, wiped out. Depending on how well I did, determined if or when I would be comfortable enough to try again. It became a fun measurement of healing successes. Well, at least for me, anyway.

Any small gain in any area of my health maintained my encouragement and confidence to try more things. I tried doing everything I thought I could handle, either alone or with some assistance. If it was too risky, I bowed out. Eventually, I tried more eye-hand-coordination sports, very easy walking trails, practiced driving, and riding my racing trike. I am grateful for improvements accomplished more than twenty years later, especially regaining sensations in my limbs, temperature, near-normal walking ability without devices (I call it free walking), and coordination of movements, particularly eye-hand reactions. I hope I make the case that improvement may occur at any point post-stroke through true efforts and continually doing your best to maintain an upbeat, confident frame of mind.

•• ● ••

Visualization is another recovery therapy that helps the brain rewire after a stroke by triggering neuroplasticity the same way physical practice does. Maura became an excellent track athlete, initially as a sprinter for her private track club, then mid-distance for high school and college teams. I visualized us running marathons and 10K charity races together, I visualized continuing to run with Alan in additional charity events with hopes of finishing the race before him. On those few occasions I was able to stay close to Alan, we would sprint to the finish line, seeing who had the last bit of *juice* left to edge out the other. It would have been so very special to me if Maura and I could have shared those opportunities together. Visualizing our running together gave me hope that one day my dream may come true. I visualized playing softball with Sara the way Edward and I did whereby the batter held the softball and then lofted it straight up in the air with hopes of timing our swing such that the ball was hit into the outfield so the other could catch it.

Jennifer was a champion field hockey player, so all I could visualize was me watching another ball be hit into the goalie box. I so much wanted to be re-involved in my Girlies' sports worlds. With Eldon, it would have been boxing, but I already suffered one brain injury, so my visual thoughts were short lived. The point is *visualization* helped me get through the tougher parts of recovering.

I might have had a chance to keep up with Maura. I playfully gave her a nickname of *Run Like Wind* because she was fast. I joked one year that I had a chance to beat her when several years later, Maura had surgery on her legs and was using crutches for several days. One afternoon, I saw her at the top of the stairs about to make her way down, a routine Maura mastered easily carrying crutches in one hand, while holding the banister with the other. I remembered my negotiation of stairs and asked if I could help her in some manner. Maura politely declined, and before I could blink, she came tumbling down the stairs at lightning speed, crashing into the front door! As horrific as it was to see Maura's body bounce around on the stairs, she was perfectly fine, and we both laughed hysterically out of relief and irony! Joking at these moments adds levity. Attempts at humor are healthy for me.

Art therapy as an active part of recovery continues gaining strides in its role to assist stroke survivors. "Art therapy enriches lives through the use of art making and the creative process. It can be used to improve anything from cognition to self-esteem and emotional support. It is especially effective for those with difficulties with communication and expressing themselves, which is often one of the challenges people have after a stroke" (American Art Therapy). It can be a useful tool in assisting rehabilitation therapies and reconnecting mind and body. It is also a useful tool in "providing an outlet of self-expression for non-verbal survivors."

My daughter, Jennifer, an art therapist states,

> Art has a beautiful way of communicating feelings when it seems impossible to verbally articulate them." Further explaining, "Art therapy is a unique modality that can be incorporated in mental health treatment for people of all ages and conditions. Art therapy integrates different creative processes and materials tailored to each client's goals established in counseling. It is a fascinating way of exploring our subconscious and is a less intimidating way of processing feelings especially related to trauma. It is an optional experience that can be offered in conjunction with traditional talk therapy utilizing the creative process to explore self-expression and improve overall well-being.

By my five-year stroke anniversary, I was very fortunate to have achieved many major recovery milestones. I appreciated newfound physical strengths, body coordination, dissipated brain fog, slight relief from constant dizziness, and other things. Now nineteen-plus years out, I still eagerly participate in varying rehabilitation exercises, including cognitive and physical therapies, enabling myself to continue healing, and have greater confidence in my ability to accomplish things I thought were no longer possible. I exercise walk two or three days a week and weight train another two or three days a week. If I have completed the six-day regimen, I rest my body on the seventh day or do something less strenuous. I rarely drive for safety reasons, plus it is just not as enjoyable. Nor is my ability to sit for a long time enjoyable because sitting for too long brings about periodic legs spasms. When I do elect to drive, I always jokingly tell my passengers to wear the helmet I passed out to them, and tell people if they don't like how I drive, then stay off the sidewalk, as the saying goes!

I viewed a TED Talk at our support group meeting. TED stands for Technology, Entertainment, and Design. TED TALKS are today considered the three broad subject areas collectively shaping our world and showcasing important research and ideas from all disciplines and exploring how they connect. TED Talks are promoted as saying they are dedicated to researching and sharing knowledge that matters through short talks and presentations informing and educating global audiences in an accessible way (*Google*).

One afternoon I was alone and so bored! I scored major brownie points when I decided to clean the kitchen refrigerator. Not just the shelves, bins, and freezer compartment, but I also wiped down the sticky jars and checked every sell by date! Abbey almost fell in love with me again!

This TED Talk showcased a stroke survivor presenting his personal recovery journey. He believes he is now living his second life. His first life ended at age thirty-nine, the age at which he suffered his stroke. He struggles to understand his perceptions against the reality he now faces, stating his best therapy is trying to live each day normally and to do things he could not even accomplish yesterday and count those as victories.

Many days after my daily out-patient rehabilitation exercises were finished, Abbey would drop me off at the house to run her errands plus those on behalf of the family. I quickly became bored if not productive between the hours of my Girlies returning home from school and Abbey finishing all errands. Reading was still difficult, but my vision slowly continued to mend. Simple things brightened my day. I was not able to drive yet, so running errands with Abbey quickly became my favorite pastime because I could *leave the four walls of our house* and do something different. I missed the freedom and productivity running errands gave me, so I wasn't picky where we went. Pick a mundane chore, and I was happy. My happiest drives were to attend my Girlie's weekend or weeknight sporting events and practices. Those times perked me up the most.

Nearly twenty years later, I remain self-conscious about how I walk and of scars remaining from procedures necessary to place the feeding tubes and of other wounds on my face. My medical charts paint a terrible picture of me if you never met me. During an office visit at a practice I have never visited, a doctor entered the exam room, and within seconds, she very politely said to me, "You look amazing; from reading your chart, I expected to see a patient much, much worse given what you have been through." I took her comment as a compliment.

I received an insurance rejection notice recently for Long Term Care stating, "At this time, we cannot offer you insurance." Then, blah, blah, blah, with a closing salutation that my hopeful insurance agent and I laughingly interpreted as, "He is lucky to be alive and fully functional." We both knew the gist of what the company was conveying *between the lines*, even though they found a way to write a declining letter professionally. After we *pulled ourselves together*, the prospective agent asked if I wanted to appeal. I said, "The company is not wrong, so I do not take exception." We shared another hearty laugh.

Chapter 18:
Controlled Responses

I consider myself to be constantly healing because my recovery journey is not over. Looking back, I still struggle to understand why I had little control over my anger despite so much medical reading, research, and help. Much of what I read boiled down to the brain would heal when it's ready with tips on how to help yourself using time, patience, rest, exercise, healthy foods or supplements, and completing varying cognitive therapies. These were stressed as a means to help. But, when my behavior was destroying family bonds, I found time to be against me, not a luxury to wait for things to correct and rewire.

My thoughts toward helping myself was a simple process to grasp. If you know your actions are wrong or unacceptable, then STOP IT! It is my responsibility to end my negative behaviors. Others can offer help and hope, but it is my responsibility to stop hurting us, my family. I could not comprehend having little control over my emotions, frequently asking myself how much of my problem was me and how much was my brain? I would not accept my brain injury was in complete control, and with time and patience, things would dissipate and resolve themselves. My brain accounted for what I thought was a small part of the broader equation. Yet, I read and consulted with doctors who confirmed the brain is indeed that powerful, sometimes needing mental health assistance to get back on track to return to our normal.

Eventually, I pursued private mental help assistance, hoping to learn coping strategies and mitigate environmental stressors compounding my anger. I also sought other help by attending my faith's sabbath services to feel spiritually connected to God beyond my heart and mind. I desired God's healing help, and I needed to be understood; I needed to be *me* again. I was *sick* of myself. Looking in the mirror was upsetting to see my face but not me. I woke up most days wanting to do activities that made us happy and *normal*. Of course, some days I was more successful than other days because all of us were walking on eggshells, wondering when things would turn ugly rather than focusing on the positive moment.

I exhausted strategies, words of advice, and any rational means to end or at least filter my verbal anger. Again, I was wrong. I am not hiding behind my stroke. It was a daily fight with myself to take a deep breath and count to ten before staunchly defending myself on issues I believed were being dismissed or discounted by my family. JW also said in the interview, "Who I am post-stroke still matters."

I still mattered and thought I was protecting myself, which only poured salt on an open wound, as the saying goes. Friends reminded me to ask myself, "Is defending yourself truly worth it? It is a non-starter, certainly not worth the damage you are causing."

Agreed. Most times, I should have remained quiet because my misguided actions only made things worse although that was not my intent. Feeling dismissed led to removing myself from the equation rather than stirring up trouble. It became easier to accept conversations flowing without my participation; that was the better choice versus negatively lashing out and wishing I had not said *that* or wishing I could take *that* back. I should have apologized more, but my family's probable thought was for me to stop apologizing and end our nightmare. I rarely found a successful route toward a productive result, so I resolved to remain silent as much as possible to mitigate my irrational anger and frustration.

My coping skills felt as if each day was a new learning experiment, evaluating what worked yesterday and seeing if I could apply that response today. I coped through hope and reason that I would somehow magically change. It was at this stage I finally sought help, even though it was way past when I should have first reached out. I was at least cognizant of my impulsive behaviors and constantly worked to end them and become a better person. That was the first step toward ending my negative behaviors.

Maintaining appropriate control or formulating a means to avoid hypersensitive negative behaviors was the most challenging. I had to focus energy on thinking before responding, pausing before reacting, and allowing myself time to decide the most appropriate response. Taking time to pause and actually think about how to react felt new to me, as if I never learned this approach back in elementary school and never applied it before in life's situations. I was again taught something I had known all my life. What I was doing for so long post-stroke was impulsively blurting out responses then wishing I never said this or that, and after the fact thinking, *I call it rather than taking a moment to formulate an appropriate response first.* That would have been a better choice, likely avoiding the. pitfalls of irrational, impulsive, angry behaviors. Pausing a moment to think about how to react was, indeed, an effective way to navigate situations and identify my trigger points for overreacting. Slowly, I achieved far greater control over my behaviors, leading to more thoughtful and constructive responses and opening productive communication.

As the years march forward, these behaviors have dissipated significantly, though. Periodically, I slip up when emotions overtake my head faster than rational thought can prevail. If I am overly passionate or protective of a particular matter, a person's purposeful disregarding, discounting, or attacking attitude toward my actions or thoughts will make me verbally angry and highly defensive. I remain very open-minded and welcoming of opinions, just not when attacking or known to be factually wrong. Pre-stroke I could filter responses more reasonably. Sometimes, if I am overstimulated or tired, I can have a momentary flare-up, and I go into my unfiltered mode. I do my best to recognize my mistake and apologize quickly, consciously reminding myself not to slip backward, trying to stay my better-healed *self*.

Today, I am more rational, and anger is now replaced by daily reminders of how fortunate I am and have been to reach varying new phases of life over the past twenty years, as in watching my Girlies successfully progress in their lives, their hopes and dreams or enjoying my active retirement life by spending more time with family and friends and the greatest joy of being grandfather, or as we say, "Geepa!"

Chapter 19:
Sleep

My primary neurologist constantly reinforced the critical need for rest and sleep after a stroke and suggested sleep study tests to measure the quality of sleep I was receiving to maximize recovery efforts. It was also suggested I rest about ten minutes per hour initially, something impossible to do once I returned to work on a regular basis. I wanted to rest but ALWAYS FEARED being seen as weak, shirking my responsibilities, or seen as a lazy non-contributor. However, I very quickly learned to fit in these breaks as much as possible because otherwise, indeed, my brain told me IT IS TIME TO REST.

I would become impatient, anxious, and therefore, my quality of work suffered. At home, if I did not rest periodically. I had mood swings or grew frustrated and impatient. My neurologist firmly believed in resting and suggested closing my office door, dimming the lights, reducing surrounding stimulation, and refreshing my brain and reducing stress during these moments to help with proper recovery.

I was usually mentally exhausted after work and over-stimulated by noise and the normal daily work. By the time I returned home for the evening, I was functioning on low energy, trying to help with normal family activities and responsibilities. I tried to help with homework, although my Girlies would tell you I could not help them much after their finishing fourth grade, and that would be a true assessment! I tried being a sous chef for Abbey, or at least my version of one, while she prepared delicious healthy meals for the family. I, or the Girlies set the table and then helped to clear the table after dinner and any other cleanup of dishes etc. I was often unusually tired and did not understand why given my very active lifestyle.

I was repeatedly told by my doctors, neurologists, nurses, and rehabilitation experts that after a stroke, your brain and body soak up so much energy while healing especially immediately following the event. At the current stroke support group I now attend, we had a neurologist guest speak followed by a typical question and answer segment. With his doctor-supported research that states frequent resting, he differentiated between rest and sleep, which enhances the patient's ability to learn and then store and retrieve that information or memory. For me, resting helped ensure I had the alertness to learn and participate in new therapy exercises especially during exertions of learning how to walk again.

Numerous sources of research state fatigue is very common after any type of stroke or transient ischemic attack (TIA) with sometimes lingering effects lasting years after the stroke event. This fatigue on-set can present itself at any time after a stroke and is not a *normal* tiredness that does not necessarily improve with rest. Nearly everyone I have met at a support group or brain injury charity event or spoken to about their concerns, have complained of frequent needs or desires to shut down and rest. "This is because the brain requires extra energy to heal the damage, leaving less energy available for typical functions such as staying alert. While the brain normally uses twenty percent of the body's total energy, that percentage increases during the first few weeks to months following a stroke"(National Library of Medicine). "Therefore, in order for the brain to be able to achieve an optimal recovery, individuals must have adequate amounts of quality sleep."

Once home, I found myself becoming easily tired as I tried my best to keep up with everyday events and the bombardment of *normal household life* stimuli. My desire to sleep, or at least rest, had everything to do with my healing brain and nothing to do with laziness. I felt as though Abbey forgot how active I was pre-stroke, and my Girlies only knew who I am now. They see a tired father struggling and unpleasant to be around. Of course, they could not see my former self as very active participating in charity running events and marathons with my brother, Alan, weight training either alone or with Edward, or me with Alan and Eldon at a community gym trying to prove their little brother could still defend himself! I played in adult recreation basketball leagues with Eldon and was very proud of myself for keeping fit and healthy. As time marched on, Abbey and I and the Girlies would biker ride together, play basketball, or enjoy other sports together. Once a year, Abbey and I participated in a formal bike/pedal tour across Maryland. One year, Jennifer, then age nine, joined us via a tandem bike with Abbey.

Not realizing so much rest is required after a stroke, it never occurred to me why I was so tired. I was fortunate to lead a healthy lifestyle pre-stroke, so I did not understand how a stroke slowed me down so much. When I finally asked doctors, I was told the extra need for rest was a byproduct of my stroke and to rest often, and take the time to heal properly. Quite frankly, I was ashamed of resting from time to time and still worried about being viewed as weak or less than an equal supporter on any *front*, in any manner, let alone miss a pleasurable activity with my family.

Chapter 20:
Durable Medical
Equipment

The folks at *Flint Rehab* advise that patients need a consistent, strong home therapy regimen. The patient should work together with doctors and his/her therapy team to receive post-stroke exercises for your unique needs and abilities. As you know, each person will need to assess his/her home variables. Costs may become a factor as there may be needed medical equipment and costs associated with those, as well as any in-home rehab.

To help ensure you and your family's comforts and requirements are met, the American Stroke Association "suggests having your home evaluated for safety and comfort ideally before returning home. Assess your needs, preferences, and abilities as well as the existing features of your home."

In terms of in-home caregiving, specific to cost, I have learned of opportunities to mitigate stress when a survivor or the family requires caregiving assistance. One opportunity offers the possibility of having a nursing student provide home help in exchange for a room or room and board, providing a win-win scenario for the student and family. The student obtains valuable, real-life experience working with a patient. The family receives a level of care in a manner that perhaps is more affordable and convenient.

While in the three hospitals, a couple of nurses shared with me that some of them are interning or are a traveling nurse who welcome affordable housing while in town working or trying to settle in. The hospital assists greatly with their necessary planning and arrangements, but other options areappreciated. This may be a potential avenue to explore for those looking at possible and different opportunities for home health care.

Durable Medical Equipment (DME) is typically designed for home therapeutic use and may be an option beyond the traditional means of obtaining therapy once discharged. *Flint Rehab* writes, "Seventy percent of stroke survivors need more therapy than what their insurance covers. Therapist's time can be too expensive." Although patients often go to outpatient therapy afterward, this is not a long-term solution for most because survivors may not have adequate therapy care or days remaining on his/her insurance approvals upon returning home. DME may be a less costly alternative, and a patient does not have to disrupt their consistent exercise program by continually obtaining insurance approvals. No breaks in exercise therapy may provide maximum chances of faster recovery."

In another article entitled, "Tools to Spark Recovery Tips," it states,

> Consistent rehabilitation is key in speeding up your recovery results. When the brain has consistent stimulation through regular practice you reinforce and strengthen the newconnections in your brain faster, which will have you seeing faster results. So be sure to stick to your regimen! When you are not continuing this intense rehab after discharge to home, you will likely plateau or even lose what function you had previously reclaimed."

Sometimes, computer software may provide therapies. Here are some ideas that may become predominate in the years to come.

- Devices for hands or ankles to monitor flexibility, dexterity, mobility, and strength.
- Programmed devices to be interactive with the patient and provide real-time results, statistics, evaluations, guidance, and feedback.
- Data via devices that can be provided via phone or tablet.

My balance remains unsteady, though it has significantly improved over the years. I am very fortunate that my needs are minimal, but I periodically complete formal outpatient therapy to tweak and improve my balance concerns as needed. As mentioned, I will occasionally dust off my cane. I have assisted devices for shower rails and a built-in tile seated bench, which, thank goodness, I rarely use except for the convenient placement of my body wash and shampoo.

I might have a slight advantage when I become an older gentleman with a potential need for assisted devices in my daily activities because I have learned at a younger age how to use a cane, quad cane, walker, and wheelchair.

Chapter 21:
Socializing

Socializing was sometimes uneasy for me, depending on the venue and my mood because I was often overtired and irritable. Noisy places forced me to strain my voice over the crowd, so I could somewhat be heard. Most times I whispered into Abbey's ear what I wanted to say to someone, and she then spoke for me. If she were not with me, I had to be very close to the person I was speaking with, or worse, I tried to practically whisper into the person's ear. Perhaps, it seemed funny at first but having a conversation with someone must have some boundaries. Mints or gum were on my person most all times. I became selective of where and when I went out as it took a good deal of mental and physical energy to prepare myself to go out in my best health. Thank goodness friends and family understood and even became familiar with my facial expressions or gestures to communicate without straining my voice. Most all my conversations were short and to the point, using just enough words to convey my response. When I finally was allowed to have vocal cord surgery, I was able to produce improved and louder vocal sounds, but my left vocal cord remained paralyzed. Speaking on the phone is my greatest challenge because I still suck in air after several words causing an unintended slurring of words or a need to stop talking between thoughts because of feeling light-headed. The person listening on the other end of the phone cannot read my lips or see my body language to fill in any missed words.

Some days I didn't even want to be with myself, so why would others want to be with me? I would jokingly say to myself. At the beginning of my recovery, I lost a couple of good friends because I had difficulty socializing and keeping my anger in check. In addition, I had to ask for assistance to lift, carry, or move things more times than I care to count. I was relearning how to walk and would stumble, maybe take an occasional light fall even while using a walker or cane, so I limited social outings with friends out of potential embarrassment. I remain subconscious of needing assistance from time to time, so I may not *go out* if I think I may need help walking or have trouble swallowing food as I still choke because my throat muscles are weak. It is quite the dramatic scene when I have an occasional choking event. My friend, Jeff, uses his joke, "I have the nine and the one already dialed; do you need me to dial the other one?" Just for that comment, I will pass out and fall on his bike next time! Getting in and out of a vehicle, especially when dizzy, *has humorous moments.* Thank goodness, I have a great circle of friends who gladly help me, and do not care about any potential mishap—"Just get out and enjoy," they always say.

Chapter 22:
Returning to Work

I regarded performing any ADL as therapeutic mentally and physically because I was working to accomplish something. "Just doing life," I coined. Simply showering and getting dressed faster and better was a win. When I returned to work, the daily work, teamwork, and camaraderie exercised my brain. I pushed myself hard to return to *my normal,* and a great part of *my normal* was my working career.

I missed work, friends, colleagues, and the brain stimulation of participating in daily decision making for ongoing activities. I loved my career and felt relevant. I missed teamwork interactions, teaching future generations of leaders, and having them teach me the latest technologies. Going back to work signified the next levels of my fortunate, successful recovery. An online article, "9 Reasons You Should Return to Work After Stroke" states, "Research suggests that a lack of activity can contribute to mood disorders. This is because being idle can lead to feelings of isolation, boredom, and a lack of purpose, all of which can negatively impact mental health."

"Keeping your mind active is an important component of recovery from a stroke. Going back to work after a mild stroke, once you're ready, can be mentally stimulating," says Einor Ben-Assayag, a senior researcher in the neurology department at Tel Aviv Sourasky Medical Center in Tel Aviv, Israel."

After three-and-a-half months of at-home recovery and outpatient rehabilitation services, I started the mental process of returning to work and moving forward with additional normalcy and life routines I enjoyed. I still had the ability to continue working in my capacity as a manager and leader, desiring to impart my wisdom to bring up the younger generation of leaders. I wanted to continue traveling overseas, including war zones, if approved. Logistically, there were many details to arrange and sew up, beginning with opening other discussions with doctors, my family, and career service personnel. A few friends and family members politely asked me to consider going out on disability, fearing I was placing undue pressure on myself for desiring to work again. While I appreciated their suggestions and reasoning, I never gave their suggestions any sincere consideration, not because of pride as one friend voiced. Instead, it was because I was healing and absolutely knew I still had so much more to contribute. I am thankful my career service felt the same way, and I was grateful to be welcomed back after I passed all medical tests, allowing me to continue my domestic and overseas duties.

My neurologist and work doctors approved my return to work with a few considerations. One implemented plan had me start working part-time, then gradually increase my hours each week. My neurologist's approval allowed me to cross a big hurdle and proudly reach another huge milestone toward full recovery. Now, the heavy logistical considerations of transitioning back to work had to be *ironed out*. Once back at work, my morning routine required additional time to prepare for the day. Rise and shine began at 4:30 AM with a shower. Fortunately, at this point, I did not require as much assistance to complete my rituals, but the few times I needed help, waking Abbey at that hour was playfully risky. Getting dressed was often entertaining because I still had diminished feelings in my arms and hands, so tying my dress shoes sometimes was a frustrating production until dress loafers entered my world—problem solved!

I got a *kick* out of trying to button my dress shirts or tying my necktie into something other than a noose on days I felt sorry for myself. My Girlies provided some dressing assistance, and Abbey and a couple of work colleagues drove me to work until it was safe for me to begin driving again. Returning to work was a tremendous motivator to keep pushing myself to accept more challenges, and returning to work was therapeutic stimulation for my brain. I felt I was needed again, and as a contributor to the work mission and to my family. I felt less of a family burden and more like a co-supporter.

I wanted to rearrange my office a tad to make mobility easier for me. I needed to place things frequently required in areas with easier access. I moved the things that were easy to rearrange or move. For other things, friends were kind enough to help, and everything was quickly moved into place. Later, my moderate perfection side kicked in when I realized a bookshelf was three inches off its *perfect* placement. Much to my chagrin, I took one look and said I could do that myself. Mind you, my right side is stronger than the left side, so when I moved the bookshelf, the right side moved fine; the left side was thrown into a tilt. Now, leaning too far forward, I had no strength to stop its downward motion. The bookshelf and I hit the floor in a thunderous noise. Books and body parts were everywhere. I was fine, but the bookshelf was another story. Fearing utter humiliation, I picked up my cane and got off the floor faster than I thought possible, hand brushing my suit off while acting calm and cool! The two female work colleagues in the office next door came over, saw the mess, and asked if everything was ok. "We heard the loud crash, so we fully expected to see you laid out on the floor needing mouth to mouth." Only five seconds earlier, indeed, I was on the floor. I laughed and said, "Who knew a few books could make so much noise!" I had to smirk at myself to keep from crying.

I was thankful I did not require special accommodations upon returning to work but knew it would be available if I needed assistance. I just needed to relax and trust myself much as I had before my stroke. I was anxious to prove myself worthy again, inviting humorous banter and playful *jabs* when I did require a bit of help.

One afternoon, my office division wanted to go out to lunch to celebrate the successful end of a project. We rarely acknowledged our efforts when completing projects, but this was a *different occasion.* So, we took a break and went to a restaurant. No alcohol was served, but judging by how I stepped off the curb toward my colleague's vehicle, you would not know that. I was *beyond dizzy* trying to speak to many colleagues in a noisy venue and then walking a short distance to the car. I had no sense of spatial cues, and my world spun. I did not ask for help to step off the curb, so I lost my balance a little bit; the two parked cars I was walking in between kept me propped up! The restaurant patrons looking out the window had a hardy laugh watching me. I suspect I was the highlight of their day.

•••

Abbey was my primary driver for everything, including driving me to work at 0530, dropping me off at the handicapped entrance, then picking me up several hours later. Walking from the parking lot to my office desk usually took extra time because I stopped occasionally to re-settle my dizziness and spatial cues. Once inside the building, I felt awkward being unable to keep up with others and self-conscious of how I walked, though my cane helped limit serpentine drifting. Morning rituals for Abbey and me were time-consuming from the moment I woke up to arriving at my office and her returning home, but she never complained, remaining supportive of my goals.

I was very nervous the first day in the office, not so much because of any minor cosmetic or physical deficits; those were superficial; it was the unknown expectations of how I would be treated and my fears of no longer being relevant, stereotyped, or pushed aside. I felt I could not exhibit any weakness, make any mistakes, or give any reason to doubt my leadership capabilities, so I only *took limited off-clock* breaks for a few minutes as a suggested condition of returning. These breaks were to rest and refresh my brain, so I would not *over-tax* it. Stressors could set back my progress and perhaps cause other side effects or damage. My left vocal cord remained non-functional in a total paralysis state, nor did my right vocal cord improve. I could barely speak above a whisper; anything louder required an exhausting physical effort of sucking in air to produce audible sounds, which made my voice extremely breathy, raspy, and me dizzy. I was concerned about not having credibility because of my extremely weak voice and how I had to manage air flow in a very deliberate manner. I feared being dismissed or minimized at office or higher-level meetings if I did not appear strong enough or took too long to convey my viewpoints. Colleagues who knew me pre-stroke playfully joked, saying my new voice was *sexy* or that they missed my former powerful, husky, baritone Barry White singer's voice. I had none of those adjectives but enjoyed the banter. At times, I indeed found myself processing previous sentences while others moved on or conversed in rapid, back-to-back exchanges.

Beyond the love of my job, I greatly desired to equally provide my Girlies with a solid head start on their future ambitions, enjoy family vacations, and for Abbey and me to eventually be able to enjoy a modest retirement. Now, I needed to fulfill my desire to be a contributing income earner. We were so very grateful we never lost any income during my recovery because I was prudent in saving my sick- days-time-off. In addition, I was healthy for most of my working career, allowing me to continually save time and carry it forward. Therefore, we were not burdened with immense financial pressures because I had plenty of paid sick leave time off to sustain our normal income.

In preparation for workdays, every evening before going to bed, I used my mortar and pestle to grind and crush medicines into powder, then packaged and prepared it for mixing with my tube-fed bolus for my morning feeding break at work. One morning, I was feeling quite weak, so I decided to have my breakfast of champions at home minutes before being picked up by a work colleague. My decision set off a sequence of embarrassing events rather quickly.

Whenever I was being picked up, I looked out the front door several minutes before my colleague's arrival and waited. Since I decided to *tube feed,* I was sitting at the kitchen table, having forgotten to open the door and turn on the porch lights. Instead, I was at the table with my shirt partially hanging out from my suit, my feeding tube partially exposed, and my pants somewhat open to access the valve. Moments later, the doorbell rang. I panicked and yelled loudly for Abbey to please open the door and let my colleague inside. Well, Abbey is a sound sleeper and did not hear me. In full reaction mode and not thinking, I abruptly stood up to answer the door while yelling for help and also trying to alert my colleague that I was coming to open the door. Now, if you are unfamiliar with a feeding tube, my sudden movements caused a volcanic reaction inside the tube, and the liquid feed reversed course. The liquid content splashed out from the top of the tube onto my shirt and floor. All *this* happened before I reached the door; my left hand held the tube, while my right hand ensured my suit pants stayed up. Then, when I reached for the doorknob, I stood before her in my cartoon boxers. After that incident, Abbey began driving me to work until I passed a scheduled driver's course to drive again.

••●••

While I was tube feeding at work, I always closed my office door, which is very rare as I make myself available to staff at any time. In the back of my mind, I was slightly concerned a moment would arrive when someone may need to speak with me during tube feeding. In those instances, I requested staff knock before entering; otherwise, they entered at their own risk. I would let folks know I was tube feeding, so they should call or knock first before visiting. I sometimes put a sign on my door that read, "Enter at Your Own Risk" or "Please Do Not Disturb." Colleagues gave me "Do Not Disturb" signs they'd taken from a variety of hotels as a joke.

Each day built greater confidence in maintaining my personal and professional self-esteem and trusting myself to have a confident game face. Fortunately, everyone was very welcoming. The greatest amount of credit toward achieving my return to work goes to Abbey and my Girlies. Those first few weeks back at work were very tiring both mentally and physically but very rewarding because it further secured my thankfulness for what I still have, keeping me grounded and appreciative for what I was able to regain. I was in better health because of so many caring people and my reaffirming of God's blessings. Returning to work was not the end of my recovery. I still had a great deal to mentally and physically overcome. My return was a welcome milestone, serving as a positive catalyst to never let go of hope. I worked another fifteen-plus years, completing a most wonderful thirty-three-plus year career! Sure, some assignments were better than others, but I happily acknowledge I am grateful for my career and service to our country. I was given every opportunity I desired. Post-stroke, I had to maintain self-awareness that there were some assignments I could no longer accept or compete for, and while it was difficult for my ego to accept, I never felt slighted. It was all about self-awareness. Sometimes, I chose to gracefully bow out from accepting an assignment or competition rather than place health risks on myself and, most importantly, any type of risks on others.

Chapter 23: Forgiveness

My stroke was not seeded in a one-time event, hopefully never to occur again. Instead, it represented a continuation of the damage I inflicted on my family and my worrying if I would have another one as I age. Those concerns are the toughest to silence, but I try to always listen to my neurologist who said, "Accept you had a stroke, and move on without worrying and being scared." The Stroke Foundation wrote an extensive article on their website entitled, "You are Now in Recovery and Will Be Continuously Working on your Recovery for the Rest of your Life." Indeed, this is precisely how I feel as I continue learning and improving. I am lucky and pleased with where I am now, though my efforts to become *whole again* are not finished as I set out to define who I am now and ask for forgiveness.

Forgiving yourself means different things to each of us. The Mayo Clinic wrote an online article entitled, "Take steps to feel better about yourself." Under the subtitle, "Adjust your thoughts and beliefs," one suggestion involves forgiving yourself and recognizing everyone makes mistakes. "Mistakes aren't permanent reflections on you as a person." They're moments in time. Tell yourself, "I made a mistake, but that doesn't make me a bad person." Indeed. Part of forgiving myself is recognizing and balancing all the positive changes and things I have accomplished before and after my stroke and acknowledging the valued goodness I have provided my family, friends, and those less fortunate. Forgiving myself means reflecting upon a portion of my past I wish to forget forever.

I still have not forgiven myself for the stress and damage I caused my family and my failure to be a role model, so I am stuck in my past unable to let go of my gut-wrenching battle between regret and guilt-ridden moments as I look back at that time and try desperately to make peace with the emotional mistakes I made and caused my family. I will never get that time back again. There is no *re-do*. While the stroke did not kill me, the shame and guilt I still feel because of my behaviors is worse. My sister-in-law, Ruth, elegantly summed up that time as, "You were never intentionally ugly; you were living with a hell inside you while desperately trying to find your normal self. Your life was torn apart. People should gracefully understand your brain was traumatized and not hold anything against you during that awful time. Forgive yourself. Don't forget about forgiving yourself." As I try forgiving myself, I try listening to others who have said people need to understand your brain injury controlled you, so your resulting behavior was not you.

Ruth, friends, psychologists, neurologists, and survivors I have interviewed regarding their recovery and those I met at brain injury survivor events all offered a common denominator, saying my stroke diminished control of my rational mind. I was not myself during that time. I counter their thoughtful reasoning with I did not hurt just myself; I hurt my family. If I were the only person affected, I could move forward. I suspect Abbey and my Girlies chose to find closure by putting this chapter of life behind them, moving forward in their manner and time with or without necessarily forgiving me.

An acquaintance, who is a priest, texted me a passage stating, "Failure is a process. We will sometimes fail in our endeavors and challenges.

Accept the failures, deal with them, and keep moving forward." This passage may or may not be his own words, but it is a thought-provoking statement. Regardless of whom I spoke to, what I read, the presentations I attended or listened to via social media, or during my times of introspection, little helped. Eventually, I looked to my religious faith for comfort and hopeful answers. While all avenues provided helpful insights and understanding, finding the breakthrough answer that assists with forgiving myself remains challenging.

My interpretations from reading various Bible scriptures or speaking with clergy and religious friends ask that we repent our sins and ask God for forgiveness. God will then unquestionably forgive our transgressions even if we led or are leading a less-than-respectable life and asking for forgiveness on a deathbed situation. Clergy have told me to help heal, I should provide charitable giving to those in need. I am proud that since I was a young adult, I often helped others, however possible, by paying good deeds forward. I learned of this concept through Uncle Solomon and from my parents. As a young boy and early teenager, it started with shoveling snow for others, watching Mom making dinner, or going grocery shopping for a neighbor who was laid up in bed sick. Or there was Dad investing his time on neighborhood projects and acting as a community activist. Watching them and others do good deeds taught me to do the same when possible.

The 2000 movie, *Paying It Forward*, is about a boy attempting to make the world a better place by doing good deeds for others after his social studies teacher gives his class an assignment. The boy hopes his good deeds are then passed on to others who, in turn, continue passing the kindness to more and more people. It was hoped the wide-spread kindness would change circumstances for others. The movie rekindled my focus to continue helping others and a means for me to recognize all friends and neighbors, even strangers, that helped me and my family with kind words and deeds. I feel it is my honor and polite obligation to help others, EVEN MORE SO today. I cannot thank every person who helped me, but I can certainly pay their love forward by continuing to help others. I do my best to extend kindness, especially to those in need. Now, using a term from the card game Black Jack, I try to *double-down* on efforts of kindness as our world becomes scarier and scarier and perhaps as an atonement for the unintended infliction of emotional pain I caused my family during my worst days of recovery.

Most people fret about forgiving others, not themselves. Jennifer said, "I cannot wait until my son is old enough to understand manners and for me to teach and instill kindness and politeness in him. We will change this world one child at a time."

Occasionally, I take time to acknowledge my good deeds without fanfare, but God will decide my fate of having the ability to forgive myself, hopefully by using a positive balance of all the good I try to do in life and did, especially when overseas. In conversations with religious friends from varying faiths, I believe our different religions appear to have a commonality of when a person is sincere in having remorse and the desire to change and repent. Then God is forgiving. I hold myself accountable for the anguish and turmoil I caused Abbey, Jennifer, Maura, and Sara, still not accepting it was my damaged brain as solely responsible no matter how powerful or damaged my brain became. Abbey reminds me to let go. "It is the only way you can begin healing; let go, forgive yourself, forgive the past situation, and realize it is over. Now move forward."

Country singer, song writer, George Strait has a song entitled, "Let it Go." Though not at all a song about forgiveness, its lyrics have value in other **ways** for me. In a conversation with a mental health representative, she used the term self-compassion, saying, "Bryan, have some self-compassion. Be easy on yourself." The word self-compassion defines itself, I believe, but curiosity led me to search for more substances.

Dr. Kristen Neff an *Associate Professor of Human Development and Culture, Educational Psychology Department, at the University of Texas at Austin* writes online, at self-compassion.org, It is found on the home page and states self- compassion Is simply the process of turning compassion inward. We're kind and understanding rather than harshly self-critical when we fail, make mistakes, or feel inadequate. We give ourselves support and encouragement rather than being cold or judgmental when challenges and difficulties arise in our lives. Research indicates that self-compassion is one of the most powerful sources of coping and resilience we have available, radically improving our mental and physical well-being. It motivates us to make changes and reach our goals not because we're inadequate, but because we care and want to be happy.

In another paragraph of Dr. Neff's self-compassion page, it is also described as, "Instead of mercilessly judging and criticizing yourself for various inadequacies or shortcomings, self-compassion means you are kind and understanding of yourself when confronted with your failings—after all, who ever said you were supposed to be perfect?" Further stated, Dr. Neff wrote,

> Things will not always go the way you want them to. You will encounter frustrations, losses will occur, you will make mistakes, bump up against your limitations, fall short of your ideals. This is the human condition, a reality shared by all of us. The more you open to this reality and work with it instead of constantly fighting against it, the more you will be able to feel compassion for yourself and your fellow humans in the experience of life.

I understand I cannot go back in time and change the past, but hopefully, my sincere good deeds and kindness, past and present, are reminders of the good person I am and always have been. Unfortunately, there is nothing that will erase what happened to us. I am still trying to make sense of what happened to us, learn how to welcome the present, and make a choice of not allowing that blip on the screen define and control me. I accept what happened, and I am learning to live with a regretful, remorseful time for all of us that I cannot forgive myself for causing. On the bright side, I have entered exciting new phases in life; first was retirement and now God has blessed us with a new addition to my family, a grandson.... I love being a father and now a grandfather, and God has given me an opportunity to see my children become successful in life, both personally and professionally. They have qualities and attitudes I greatly admire. Moving forward will hopefully reverse some of the hurt and damage I did with my past emotional behaviors. Those years were not the true me. Yet, an unabating deficit remains my inability to have recognized early on just how powerful the brain is and that I did not seek help earlier in my journey to change or cope with my ugly *new self.*

Permitting myself to live life in the present requires me to let go of the guilt I carry. My friend Bob says, "God wants you to forgive yourself in order to further take care of the people you love and respect by honoring their love and support for you. He often tells me, "There is no rational reason not to forgive yourself. You have repented, and God has forgiven you. For those facts to have meaning, you must forgive yourself. Believe me, if I hadn't forgiven myself, I wouldn't be the person God created me to be." Others have said forgiving yourself will lead to continual healing and growth. While my friend and piano instructor, Diana, is more blunt saying, "Stop beating yourself up and get over it! You were in survivor mode. Focus on the good, not the bad."

Forgiving myself is a decision I will hopefully make with God's help. Obtaining answers on how to forgive myself, combined with the realization of a continued bright future ahead of me while watching my Girlies successes in life and the blessed expansion of my family, my grandson, will hopefully *allow me to forgive myself.* In the interim, I enjoy every family time I can get to watch our expanded family grow up. I cherish watching my grandson discover new things in life and his daily happiness and smiles! Indeed, I am trying to focus on the good and my blessings.

Chapter 24:
What is My Purpose?

In an *AARP Bulletin* article from September 2023 entitled "The Power of Purpose," author Jo Ann Jenkins writes, "It's been said that the two most important days of your life are the day you are born and the day you find out why. Finding our purpose is what guides us and gives our life meaning."

I have mentioned to nearly everyone I know—family, friends, acquaintances, clergy, or medical professionals—for whatever reason God let me survive but not just survive. I was given another opportunity to enjoy an excellent quality of life. I believe I had some divine help, but why, why me, for what purpose? Hopefully, God is looking out for all of us, and we each serve a purpose in life.

I must have the courage and attitude to positively move forward, taking charge of continuing efforts to heal and maintain what I recaptured in finding myself again. Several years ago, a former work colleague and still friend, Alex, said of having the courage to recover and of my family going through their difficulties, "We are members of a club and wear its badge whether we want to or not."

My friend Bob said, "Your purpose will be known in time; trust God's plan; don't hurt yourself by holding onto something that no longer serves any positive purpose; forgive yourself. Let go and move forward."

Yet, after all these years, I remain wondering why I survived; for what purpose was I fortunate to survive? What is my purpose for moving forward? Am I to serve a special calling? If so, what is it? How come it hasn't become clear to me? I do not regularly volunteer my time to helping food banks, homeless shelters, hospitals and on and on, so, why did I survive and not a young child or a servant of God who openly praises God's love and goodness? Why did I survive and not others? I have spent my post-stroke years trying to figure out that reason. Friends throughout the years have said I survived because I must have a purpose for living today. "God let you survive, so your survival means something."

My buddy, Jim, said to me in the middle of this philosophical conversation on our purpose in life, specifically mine, and why was I allowed to survive, "Maybe you survived because God just didn't feel like dealing with you." After that playful jab, Jim is no longer on my holiday "shop for list."

I believe my former neighbor and friend, Michele, a schoolteacher, who has since passed away from cancer, was given the gift and purpose of teaching future generations. I am positive many of the children she taught yester-year have become a better person—and a more able person in adult life because Michele touched their lives. Her life continues in the success of former students who are productive in today's society.

I often hope to be told of my own life's purpose. Did I survive such that I can continue my dreams and perhaps spread some good along the way? Maybe I should count my blessings and get on with life. Stop all this searching. Whether I obtain answers now or later, a friend said, "The reality is...the only answer is...what you feel comfortable with accepting"

I turn toward introspective thoughts, being even more appreciative of my time on earth and trying to create more treasured moments and memories with Abbey and my Girlies, my grandson, and, hopefully, more grandchildren, more generations of family, and, of course, with my friends. I guess it's alright not to know the answers as I move ahead. Years ago, I had a philosophical conversation with a former work colleague, Alex, who said of my recovery and efforts to understand the quest for my purpose, "You and your family have courage given what you all are going through...all of you are members of a club and wear its badge whether you want to or not. Make the most of your renewed time." My brother Eldon sent me the phrase of "The Seven Rules of Life" shown below:

- Make peace with your past, so it won't disturb your present...
- What other people think of you is none of your business...
- Time heals almost everything, give time...
- No one is in charge of your happiness except you...
- Don't compare your life to others, and don't judge them, you have no idea what their journey is all about..
- Stop thinking too much; it's alright not to know the answers...
- Smile, you don't own all the problems in the world....

These rules claim no single author, but the phrase, "Seven Rules of Life," may appear in various contexts; there isn't a specific book or author that claims to have originated the ideas. Rule one resonates with me.

While viewing references to living with purpose via the *American Psychiatric Association' Online* pages of research findings, I clicked on numerous links and subtopics that speak of trying to understand or make sense of one's purpose in life with results suggesting that living with purpose may increase overall mental well-being, life satisfaction, improved health, lower risks of cognitive decline, better sleep, enhanced resilience and self-esteem, and potentially increased longevity, while decreasing chances of anxiety and depression.

In a few casual conversations with other survivors, I met a person who said to me I should have adjusted my expectations of *what life should be* to *what I wanted it to be post-stroke*, saying I should have found happiness in my *new normal*. I replied, "So, you are telling me to be happy with accepting who I temporarily became? How is that possible?"

Sometimes, I felt death would have been easier than the sense of losing my family's love because of my stroke. I consider myself to be in a work-in-progress mode, making self-improvements. I look to my family, clergy, friends, strangers, books, newspapers, and magazine articles—anything that will assist me in this self-actualization effort and my quest for why did I survive? What is my purpose?

My friend, Steve, very simply tells me, "Life is like a country song. It has sad parts and happy endings, but when all is said and done, if you have tapped your feet a few times along the way, it was worth it." Not sure where he read that saying, but I like it.

Today, I feel as though I have drowned myself in guilt rather than ex-pending greater energy on creating more productive years. Abbey says, "Yeah, but you have years upon years of good things to look forward to. You need to learn to let go and enjoy what is ahead of you." Forgiving myself is a decision I will hopefully make; love your caregivers! Maybe the life rule is "Stop thinking too much. In my case means it's alright not to know my purpose at this moment. Most desired hopeful achievement is Rule Number One—Make peace with your past, so it won't disturb your present.

Chapter 25:
Talking Points

P LEASE NOTE: These talking points provide supplemental info on strokes, statistical data, as well as awareness regarding the effects of stroke. Statistical data is a snapshot in time and may change quickly or may be reported differently depending upon who is conducting the data survey. The following information is from the U.S. Centers for Disease Control and Prevention (https://www.cdc.gov/stroke/data-research/facts-stats/index.html).

1. Stroke-related costs in the United States came to nearly $56.2 billion between 2019 and 2020. Costs include the cost of health care services, medicines to treat stroke, and missed days of work.

2. Every 40 seconds, someone in the United States has a stroke. Every 3 minutes and 11 seconds, someone dies from stroke in this country.

3. Stroke is a leading cause of death for Americans.

4. Stroke risks increase with age, but strokes can—and does—occur at any age.

5. High blood pressure, high cholesterol, smoking, obesity, and diabetes are leading causes of stroke. (One in three U.S. adults has at least one of these conditions or risk factors.)

6. Northwestern Medicine reports that seventy thousand Americans under age forty-five have a stroke.

7. An Ischemic stroke is caused by a blood clot cutting off blood flow to the brain—a clogged artery. (The CDC's research reports, "About 87 percent of all strokes are ischemic.)

8. According to the American Stroke Association, "Hemorrhagic, (pronounced hem-or-aj-ick) is defined as a bleeding stroke and make up about 13 percent of stroke cases. They occur when a weakened vessel ruptures and bleeds into the surrounding brain. Blood accumulates and compresses the surrounding brain tissue (effectively cutting off oxygen to areas of the brain. The accumulated blood puts pressure on surrounding brain areas, ultimately damaging or destroying them.)

9. An Intracerebral hemorrhage (ICH) bleeds into the brain. ICHs are hemorrhage and are a devastating form of stroke characterized by bleeding into the brain parenchyma. While this form of stroke accounts for only 10 percent, its mortality remains as high as 50% at 30-days. Over the past decade, there have been significant advances in the understanding of ICH risk, potential treatments, and outcomes.

The American Stroke Association provides these acronyms **FAST** or **BE FAST** for recognizing potential stroke symptoms.

FAST	BE FAST
Face drooping	Balance
Arm weakness	Eyes
Speech difficulty	Face drooping
Time to call 911	Arm weakness
	Speech difficulty
	Time to call 911

Knowing the **signs and symptoms of stroke** is the first step to ensuring medical help is received immediately. For each minute a stroke goes untreated and blood flow to the brain continues to be blocked, a person loses about 1.9 million neurons. This could mean a person's speech, movement, memory, and so much more can be affected.

- Sudden numbness or weakness of the face, arm, or leg, especially on one side of the body.
- Sudden confusion, trouble speaking, or trouble understanding.
- Sudden trouble seeing in one or both eyes.
- Sudden trouble walking, dizziness, loss of balance, or loss of coordination
- Sudden severe headache with no known cause.
- Vomiting
- Metallic taste in mouth
- Difficulty in swallowing

"Even after surviving a stroke, you're not out of the woods, since having one makes it a lot more likely that you'll have another. In fact, of the 795,000 Americans who will have a first stroke this year, about 610,000 are first or new strokes, killing about133,000 people, 23 percent of survivors; within those survivors, over two thirds will have some type of disability (U.S. Centers for Disease Control and Prevention).

According to the American Stroke Association, stroke is the number 3 cause of death in women and kills more women than men, but men have a higher incidence of stroke according to the U.S Centers for Disease Control and Prevention, "Stroke is a leading cause of serious long-term disability, reducing mobility in more than half of stroke survivors age sixty-five and older," and "Fewer than forty percent, maybe thirty-eight percent, of people hospitalized for stroke were younger than sixty-five."

"Problems with memory and thinking are very common after a stroke. Up to sixty percent of stroke survivors may have some type of cognitive impairment in the first year after a stroke— even experiencing dementia within three to five years post-stroke. Cognitive impairments and memory loss following a stroke are common and may affect your quality of life. This means that the way your brain understands, organizes, and stores information is affected. Problem-solving ability is usually more prevalent in stroke survivors who had a right-brain stroke. Typical cognitive problems may include

- poor concentration or attention.
- forgetfulness.
- confusion.
- inability to process information normally.
- trouble with answering questions, planning, following conversations, remembering important facts, understanding where they are, reasoning, or making judgments (American Stroke Association).

According to the CDC, 1.4 million American children and adults seek treatment for identifiable traumatic brain injuries (TBIs) from falls, car crashes, and other external blows to the head. Additionally, each year, 1 million Americans sustain acquired brain injuries (ABIs) from strokes, infections, tumors, toxins, and metabolic causes.

Although strokes frequently happen, warning signals may appear a month before a stroke. All these are known as the one-month before stroke warning signs because experiencing any of these means you need to seek medical assistance. Here are some early stroke warning signs that you shouldn't ignore.

1. Numbness or weakness: One side of the body, face, arm, or leg may experience this.

2. Confusion: Difficulty comprehending, speaking, or listening to speech.

3. Difficulty seeing: One may experience the inability to see clearly with one or both eyes.

4. Sudden difficulty walking, dizziness, losing one's balance, or a lack of coordination.

5. Sudden excruciating headache with no apparent cause.

6. One side of the face is sagging or numb.

7. One of your arms is weak or numb.

8. Speaking impairment: It refers to slurred or unusual speaking.

9. Dizziness: Balance or coordination issues or dizziness.

10. Seizures or fainting seizure or fainting.

"You don't have to be ok with it, but the quicker you accept your new reality, the quicker you can take control of it" (www.iamable.org). There are seven solid indicators you are recovering well from a stroke listed below.

1. You Make Your Best Progress Right Away

2. You Are More Independent

3. You Can Cross Your Legs

4. You Find Yourself Sleeping More

5. You Find the Need to Compensate Less with Technique

6. Your Spastic Muscles Are Twitching

7. You Have Gone Through the Grieving Process (www.iam-abble.org).

Did you know that flossing your teeth may help to lower your risk of stroke? As we know, it's a great way to remove plague around teeth that causes inflammation. This comes from a new study reported at an international stroke meeting. "A small daily habit like flossing could have significant long-term health benefits," says lead researcher Souvik Sen, M.D., professor and chair of the Neurology Department at the University of South Carolina School of Medicine. My former dentist FULLY subscribes to this belief since I first began going to his practice in 1999; he always, always, reminded me of this belief. Especially following my stroke!

EPILOGUE

In this book, I have written about topics and stories I struggled with as a stroke survivor and, hopefully, in a manner that does not come off as self-pity. I recognize I am a very fortunate survivor, who is grateful for the extra time God has given me beyond my stroke. I have seen my children (Girlies) grow up and become successful and HAPPY. And I have a new title for which I am so blessed to wear: grandfather. Suddenly, it seems I'm entering my retirement and golden years at the early age of 63.

So, allow me to leave you with this poignant poem that was written by my daughter, Maura. She writes, "It is about how I wished you could have seen the effect of the words you said." And what is my reply? Maura, with all my heart, I wish I could have seen the effect of the words I said."

LOOK DEEPER

It may seem like what you say doesn't hurt
Because I just say "ok" and nod.
But deep down beneath my surface I am hurting
That you can't see behind my false façade.

What you say builds up in my mind.
It builds and builds for a fact.
I try so hard to forget about it
But it just keeps coming back.

I am trying hard to build up enough courage to tell you.
I know I will need a lot
But I am not exactly sure how much it will take.
I just wish you could look deeper
And see that my facade is fake.

—Maura Marks

("Look Deeper" is a poem I wrote about you, Dad. This one might be hard to read. It is about how I wished you could have seen the effect of the words you said.)

Terms and Definitions

Secondary Cerebellar Stroke Effects

- **Acute cerebellar ataxia**: A sudden lack of control over voluntary movements. I experienced sudden jerky left leg movements for nearly nine months post-stroke, occurring very randomly, mostly when I continuously sat in one position for a few hours. Nothing disturbing, but when my leg decided to jerk, the movement was startling especially since there was not *a warning* beforehand.
- **Loss of coordination and balance**: This is closely related to ataxia and affects functional movements and self-care tasks.
- **Vertigo**: The feeling that the world is spinning around you. This remains problematic for me as I am dizzy nearly all the time except when I'm finally in bed for the evening.
- **Nausea and vomiting**: This effect can stem from other cerebellar stroke effects like vertigo.
- **Cerebellar cognitive affective syndrome**: This condition involves executive function, language processing, and visuospatial impairments. This can affect a survivor's mental state and behavior.
- **Impaired memory**: Cerebellar strokes can impair a survivor's working or short-term memory.
- **Difficulty with proprioception**: This refers to trouble pinpointing how your body is moving or where it is located in relation to the world around you. This indeed remains my most

difficulty. Just very recently I entered a medical building via their automatic sliding glass door. The door was still opening as I miscued and nearly banged into the door as it was still opening. The building receptionist politely held in her laughter until I said, "Go ahead! You've gotta laugh!"

- **Speech problems:** This includes conditions like aphasia or slurred speech. I do not believe I slur any words but do notice I am slightly more difficult to understand when speaking on the phone versus face to face. Occasionally, people ask me to repeat myself while conversing over the phone.
- **Eye movement disorders:** Double vision and nystagmus are common, following cerebellar stroke and can contribute to dizziness. My nystagmus remains.

The rehabilitation therapies listed below are sourced from the National Center for Biotechnology Information, National Library of Medicine. https://pmc.ncbi.nlm.nih.gov.

- *Cognitive rehabilitation therapy* focuses on restoring cognitive function through interventions or tools designed to improve memory, focus, and other cognitive skills.
- *Speech-language therapy* aims to treat difficulties with communication and language, including reading, speaking, and pragmatic communication, as well as other challenges involving movement of the tongue, mouth, and throat, such as difficulty swallowing.
- *Physical therapy* is focused on improving movement, reducing pain, and otherwise managing issues associated with mobility, balance, gait, and strength, including use of assistive devices, such as canes and wheelchairs.
- *Occupational therapy* is directed at increasing a person's ability to participate in everyday activities, including such activities of

daily living as grooming and dressing; engaging in meaningful activities; and reintegrating within the community.

- *Vocational rehabilitation* provides services to facilitate a person's ability to work or return to work and can include such services as training and job coaching.
- *Supported employment* can also be used to assist a person with significant disabilities in holding or maintaining employment to the maximum extent of their abilities.
- *Psychotherapy* and *behavior therapy* assist with cognitive, emotional, behavioral, and social-environmental challenges or barriers to community participation and adjustment to disability.

ACKNOWLEDGEMENTS

I want to acknowledge my closest buddies.

Mitchell Yockelson. Mitch has been a dearest friend of mine since infancy. I frequently seek Mitch's wise advice, especially during my difficult stroke recovery and continued healing. I always count on Mitch for his candor, perspective, blunt honesty, and guidance. Our friendship is a bond that I will forever cherish.

Gary Neuwirth. Although now with God, our endearing friendship will always remain in my heart and mind. Our shared belly laughs, life's lessons, his insights, and warm smiles are greatly missed. Gary's life was cut short, but he remains in my thoughts. I miss his physical presence, laughter, and the generous, heartfelt love and kindness he extended to my Girlies. Gary's boyish grin and eyes would beam with pride as he held and looked at his son and daughter and extended that pride to my Girlies as if they were his too. I miss Gary greatly. Until we meet again my friend!

Glenn Anderson. He is another wonderful childhood friend. His matter-of-fact *self* reminds me to learn from things while continuing to move forward. Glenn faces life straight on; throw what you want at him, and he deals with it. Then, when you least expect it, he laughs at life's journey and at himself.

Ray Dinovo. Reminds me of the faith and strength of God. He is a solid voice of reason and enriches my life with his humor, most notably, through his voice impersonations. Ray shares his thought-provoking perspectives of life and God, allowing me to remain grounded. His friendship means a great deal to me.

Nguyen Trinh. Who I admire greatly. I am thankful for his friendship and ideals of importance in life, family, and friends. He is humble with a warm, generous heart. He has proven he would "take a bullet for me."

Angelo Justiniano. For his prayers and perspectives of God's love and forgiveness. He helped me carry on through some of the most heartbreaking stories I wrote. He is my chess nemesis and master.

Jeff Dickens. For always setting the example to be your best and the best at what you do; if you are going to do something, put your best foot forward, do not slack. Jeff takes great pride in setting the bar high; he is an example for others to follow in service to our country and everyday life.

To my former neighbors, **Paul O'Donnell** and **Geoff Kemp**, for always ensuring I never slacked off on my walking rehabilitation therapies and encouraging me to remain optimistic. They dutifully ensured I walked to the mailbox daily, flanking me on both sides while making jokes or taking playful verbal jabs at me. Often, a very simple forty-five-second walk to the mailbox would often take us twenty minutes as we negotiated my walker, cane, dizziness, spatial relationships, and balance in over ninety-degree temperatures and high humidity. Paul and Geoff made a positive difference for me to keep believing in myself through humor, encouragement, and an abundance of patience, while walking with me on the hottest days of summer. Geoff moved from the neighborhood after his work with me was done, but Paul was up to the task of playfully harassing me now DOUBLE time.

To my then-community neighbors and so many friends—too many to name—thank you for supporting us, keeping us in your prayers and thoughts, making us meals, helping with driving requirements, watching over our children, creating sleepovers and social opportunities so they could have fun. Thank you for your kindness and welfare checks on me. Indeed, it does take a village!

These acknowledgments serve as my constant reminder to *pay it forward*. Thank you.

WORKS CITED

American Music Therapy Association.
www.members.musictherapy.org.

Andretta, Nicole Dr. "Emotional Resilience After Stroke." *Brain Injury Association of America.* 2025. www.biausa.org/public-affairs/media/emotional-resilience-after-a-stroke

Ben-Assayag, Einor. *Tel Aviv Sourasky Medical Center.* www.researchgate.net/profile/Einor-Ben-Assayag

"Bridge the Gap in Your Recovery." *Flint Rehab.* Aug. 2, 2024. www.flintrehab.com

Broudy, Oliver. "When Seconds Count. The Hidden Signs of a Heart Attack." *AARP.* June/July 2021. Vol.64, 4A.

Castaneda, Ruben. "9 Reasons You Should Return to Work After a Stroke." *U.S. News.* March 19, 2018. www.health.usnews.com/health-care/patient-advice/slideshows/9-reasons-you-should- return-to-work-after-a-stroke

Caswell, Jon. *Stroke Connection Magazine by American Heart Association.* Sept/Oct. 2010. www.appadvice.com/app/stroke-connecton-magazine

Caswell, Jon. "Sound Advice." *Stroke Connection Magazine.* Summer, 2013. www. appadvice.com/app/stroke-connection-magazine

Caswell. Jon. "Artful Recovery." *Stroke Connection Magazine.* Spring 2012. www.appadvice.com/app/stroke-connection-magazine

Cohen, Leonardo G. Dr. "Want to Learn a New Skill? Take Some Short Breaks." *National Institutes of Health.* April 12, 2019. www.nih.gov/news-events/news-releases/want-learn-new-skill-take-some-short-breaks.

"Community Resources for Survivors of Stroke." *Stroke Support Association.* Apr. 19, 2021. www. strokesupportassoc.org/community-resources-for-survivors-of-stroke-2

Cramer, Steven C. Dr. *Stroke Connection Magazine.* University of California, Irvine. Spring, 2012. www.uclahealth.org/providers/steven-cramer

Davis, Rick. *Between Hope and Despair: Living After a Stroke.* July 15, 2009. BookSurge Publishing. South Carolina.

Edlow, Jonathan A. "Vertigo in Cerebellar Stroke." *Stroke: Biographies of Disease.* 2008. www.Stroke Biographies of Disease 1st Edition Jonathan A. Edlow – Ebook Gate.

"Emotional and Behavioral Changes are a Common Effect of Stroke." *The American Stroke Association.* 2025. www.stroke.org/en/about-stroke/effects-of-stroke/emotional-effects

"Emotions and Stroke: Living with PBA." *Stroke Support Association.* Jan. 15, 2021. www.strokesupportassoc.org/emotions-and-stroke-living-with-pba

Fargo, Keith. "Alzheimer's Toll May Rank with Cancer, Heart Disease." *CNN.* March 5, 2014. www.cnn.com/2014/0305/health/alzheimers-deaths

Flint Rehab. "How John Recovered from Right-Side Paralysis After Stroke." Oct. 13, 2023. www.flintrehab.com/how-john-recovered-from-right-side-paralysis-after-stroke

"Generalized Anxiety Disorder, GAD." *John Hopkins Medicine.* 2025. www.hopkinsmedicine.org/health/conditions-and-diseases/generalized-anxiety-disorder

"The Healing Power of Music." *Flint Rehab.* October 16, 2023. www.flintrehab.com/healing-power-of-music

Jenkins, JoAnn. "The Power of Purpose." *AARP.* Sept. 7, 2023. www.aarp.org/advocacy/jo-ann-jenkins-power-of-purpose-2023

Johnson, Julene. "The Role of Music in Cultivating a Healthy Brain." *AARP Bulletin.* Q&A. February 2024. www.aarp.org

Josephson, Andy Dr. "Stroke 2023, A Change has Come and is Still Coming." *University of California San Francisco.* www.ucsf.edu/research.

Keegan, Carol. Fall 2013. "Stroke Connection Presents FREE Online Writing Workshop for Survivors. www.strokeassociation.org

Kim, Kyung Soo and Maichou Lor. "Art Making as a Health Intervention Concept Analysis and Implications for Nursing Interventions." *Advances in Nursing Science.* June 2022. www.journals.lww.com/advancesinnursingscience/ abstract/2022/04000/art_making_as_a_ health_ intervention__concept.6.aspx

Little, Mike. "Victim or Survivor." *Stroke Connection Magazine.* Sept./Oct. 2010. www.appadvice.com/app/stroke-connecton-magazine

Moawad, Heidi, Dr. "Personality Changes That Can Be Caused by a Stroke." *Verywell Health.* Aug. 16, 2023. www.verywellhealth.com/personality-changes-caused-by-a-stroke

"Pseudobulbar Affect." *The Stroke Foundation.* April 13, 2024. www.stroke.org/en/about-stroke/effects-of-stroke/emotional-effects/pseudobulbar-affect

Puchta, Amy E. "Recovery Tips for Stroke Survivors." *Flint Rehab.* Sept. 6, 2023. www. flintrehab.com/uploads/2022/08/Free-Ebook-Stroke-Recovery-Tips

"Rehabilitation of Therapies." *National Center for Biotechnology Information. National Library of Medicine.* www.pmc.ncbi.nlm.nih.gov

Russert, Luke. "What I Learned from My Dad." *Boston Sunday Globe Parade Magazine.* June 19, 2011. pp. 1-20. www.parade.com

Seale, Gary, Dr. "Journey of Transformation." *Brain Injury Association of America.* www.biausa.org/public-affairs/media/stroke-a-journey-of-transformation

Sen, Souvik. Dr. "Health Watch: Flossing for Heart Health and Reducing Stroke Risk." *University ofSouth Carolina, School of Medicine Columbia.* Feb. 20, 2025. www.sc.edu/study/colleges_schools/medicine/about_the_school/news/2025/souvik_sen_health_watch_flossing_study.php

"Seven Solid Indicators You Are Recovering Well from a Stroke." *I Am Able.* www.iamable.org

Shulman, Alex Kaes. "Caring for a Loved One." *Parade Magazine.* Nov. 23, 2008. parade.com/47505/parade/caring-for-a-loved-one

"The Silent Scream." *Stroke Connection Magazine by American Heart Association.* Nov./Dec. 2010. p.6. www.stroke.org

Stroke Connection Magazine by American Heart Association. Sept./Oct. 2005. www. appadvice.com/app/stroke-connection-magazine/954422817

"Take Steps to Feel Better About Yourself." *Mayo Clinic.* www.mayoclinic.org

Taylor, Jill Bolte. *My Stroke of Insight. A Brain Scientist's Personal Journey.* Penguin Random House: New York. May 26, 2009.

"Together to End Stroke." *American Stroke Association.* www.stroke.org/en/about-the-american-stroke-association/together-to-end-stroke

"Tools to Spark Recovery Tips." *Flint Rehab.* Sept. 6-8, 2023. www.flintrehab.com

"Understanding Lack of Empathy After Brain Injury and How to Cope." *Flint Rehab.* Jan. 14, 2025. www.flintrehab.com

US Centers for Disease Control and Prevention. www.cdc.gov

"What Are the Chances of Recovery from Stroke Paralysis? Exploring Studies and Methods." *Flint Rehab.* March 25, 2024. www.flintrehab.com/chances-of-recovery-from-stroke-paralysis

"2 Things Your Stroke Recovery Needs ASAP." *Flint Rehab.* www.flintrehab.com

"10 Warning Signs for Stroke You Shouldn't Ignore." *UF Health, St. Johns.* July.19, 2023. www.stjohn.ufhealth.org/news-and-blogs/2023/july/10-warning-signs-for-stroke-you-shouldnt-ignore

"15 Helpful Cognitive Rehabilitation Exercises to Sharpen Your Mind." *Flint Rehab.* Feb.15, 2024. www.flintrehab.com/cognitive-exercises-tbi

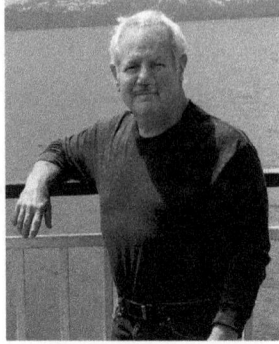

About the Author

Bryan Marks was born and raised in Montgomery County, Maryland. He graduated from Towson University in Baltimore County, Maryland, in 1984 with a bachelor's degree in business. Bryan dreams and desires were of owning a business in the hotel/hospitality industry.

He worked in the hotel/hospitality industry for three years before realizing a tremendous opportunity in 1987 to serve our great country and to fulfill a personal dream of traveling the world. Bryan married Abbey in 1989. They have three daughters, whom he affectionately calls his *Girlies*. They are Jennifer, Maura, and Sara. His Girlies are resilient, strong, accomplished, and highly talented in life and in their respective professions of licensed mental health counseling, communications/journalism, and recreational therapy, respectively.

Bryan is now a retired federal civilian employee, having completed tours in Iraq, Afghanistan, Yemen, and other regions within the Middle East and Europe over his thirty-three year-plus career. He now leads a wonderful, productive retirement life. He and Abbey reside in South Carolina and enjoy this new phase of life, learning how to play the piano, traveling, entering chess tournaments, and participating in a six-day-a-week robust exercise regimen to starve off older age.